Successful Statistics for Nursing and Healthcare

Roger Watson, Ian Atkinson &
Patricia Egerton

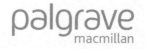

First published 2006 by
PALGRAVE MACMILLAN
Houndmills, Basingstoke, Hampshire RG21 6XS and
175 Fifth Avenue, New York, N.Y. 10010
Companies and representatives throughout the world

PALGRAVE MACMILLAN is the global academic imprint of the Palgrave Macmillan division of St. Martin's Press, LLC and of Palgrave Macmillan Ltd. Macmillan® is a registered trademark in the United States, United Kingdom and other countries. Palgrave is a registered trademark in the European Union and other countries.

ISBN-13: 978–1–4039–1652–5
ISBN 10: 1–4039–1652–7

This book is printed on paper suitable for recycling and made from fully managed and sustained forest sources.

A catalogue record for this book is available from the British Library.

10   9   8   7   6   5   4   3   2   1
15   14   13   12   11   10   09   08   07   06

Printed in China

Contents

APPENDICES

Foreword

Successful Statistics for Nursing and Healthcare is decidedly not a statistics cookbook; it helps readers to understand the concepts they are dealing with rather than simply following set instructions, and even difficult ideas are presented in a readable and accessible way. Statistics is not easy but it should be useful and enjoyable!

The authors explain the ideas underlying statistical analysis, and, through this, teach the reader how to draw valid inferences from the data they are handling. A good example of this approach is the inclusion of an introduction to probability, which of course underpins the whole area of statistical inferences (such as significance testing and confidence intervals). Throughout the rest of the book well-chosen case studies from several areas in nursing and healthcare animate the discussion, and the clear statements of objectives for each chapter signpost the learning process.

The authors have used their considerable experience in planning and analysing data from nursing and healthcare studies when constructing this book. *Successful Statistics for Nursing and Healthcare* covers all of the topics one would expect to find in a text on applied statistics and the content will appeal to a wide readership. I think it makes a very valuable addition to the literature in this field, and I am sure many readers, both students and practitioners, will agree.

Peter Jones
Professor of Medical Statistics and
Pro Vice Chancellor
Keele University

A Word About This Book

Each individual person is worth far more than any set of statistics! But for patient care in an environment of evidence-based healthcare, we must be able to use statistics – and to do so professionally means that we must understand the concepts as well as the tools of statistics. We should be able to identify the statistical techniques that help us make decisions, and also know how to avoid possible pitfalls.

So, overall, what is the secret of '*successful statistics*'? It is firstly being able *to understand statistical methods* and why they are being used, and then it is being able *to apply them competently* in appropriate situations.

In this book we include many scenarios with a nursing and healthcare focus which illustrate the use of a proper understanding of statistics. We describe the principal methods of gathering and organising data, using tables, diagrams and summaries. We look at the basic ideas underlying probability and see how they can be applied in healthcare contexts. We also introduce the main techniques by which statistics supports decision making, discussing confidence levels and different tests by which the significance of results can be quantified. By dealing with all these matters in context our hope is that Statistics is seen to be relevant, accessible and applicable.

At the front of each chapter we include a notice which highlights the chief statistical concepts covered in that chapter; this may be useful when browsing through. Alongside the text we include notices to highlight where we use examples relevant to nursing and healthcare. Several chapters contain references to books and to research papers, which are listed, together with other useful titles, in Appendix 1 'Further recommended reading' (this contains general statistics, statistics in the context of nursing and healthcare, and research papers).

An important feature of the book is the Glossary (Appendix 3), for immediate reference. It gives brief meanings of selected terms from the text and also brief explanations of some more advanced terms and techniques that may be met in professional work and in research papers.

We hope this book will help you; we wish you Success in your Statistics!

Setting the Scene

1

– *using Statistics in nursing and healthcare*

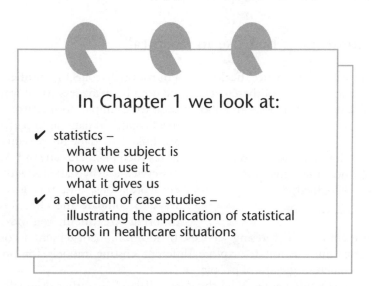

In Chapter 1 we look at:

✔ statistics –
   what the subject is
   how we use it
   what it gives us
✔ a selection of case studies –
   illustrating the application of statistical
   tools in healthcare situations

So what *is* Statistics? How is this subject relevant for people involved with nursing and healthcare? What are its basic techniques? What sort of results and conclusions can we hope to get when we use Statistics?

Well, **Statistics** tells us ways to deal with 'facts in bulk'; we might have been given these facts, known as **data**, or we might have gathered them for ourselves. Statistics helps us to organise the raw data we start with by tabulating, summarising and showing them in diagrams, so that we can use the resulting **information** to inform our planning and decision making (this area is called **descriptive statistics**). Even more importantly, it gives us methods by which we can use information from a **sample** to estimate the corresponding figures for a **population** and then to make comparisons between samples and between populations, stating the level of confidence in each result (this is known as **inferential statistics**).

1

Statistical methods should be used in just the same way that a technician uses a set of tools. Technicians deal with a range of problems by selecting and using appropriate tools from their 'kit'; similarly, various problems and challenges which healthcare professionals may face – in both practice and research – can be resolved using tools supplied by Statistics.

To illustrate some of the answers to our initial questions, we now look at a selection of 'healthcare scenarios', or case studies, which describe questions, concerns and investigations based on familiar events and requirements. We consider some of the issues involved and we show how statistical methods can be used to clarify them and to provide solutions to problems which arise. In doing this we indicate the scope of the chapters which follow in the rest of this book. We shall not be dealing with these case studies as such, but by briefly describing possible approaches we hope to encourage nurses and their colleagues to develop skills in applying Statistics.

1.1 Monitoring bed use in hospital

In their professional practice, healthcare staff routinely collect quantities of data on their patients. Some of these data can be used by managers to inform themselves of changing situations and allow them, for example, to monitor bed use in a hospital. If data on 'inpatient stay' are linked to data on patients' diagnoses then planners can study patterns of service-use by patients with different conditions, and this gives them ways to compare the effectiveness of different treatment regimes or of different methods of organising services. In addition, management accountants can use this information to explore different costing models for providing services to different groups of people.

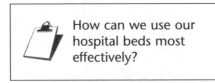
How can we use our hospital beds most effectively?

As we discuss in Chapter 2, all the data collected are either originally in the form of numbers, or else they are converted into numerical form for practical use. In this case patients' admission and discharge dates are used to calculate the length of 'inpatient stay'. This is recorded as a number, the actual number of days a patient spends in hospital. Patients' diagnoses are also usually recorded using a numerical shorthand, even though diagnoses are adjectival/descriptive. This shorthand involves a letter of the alphabet (as specified by the International Classification of Diseases, ICD, World Health Organisation, 2003). For instance, most diseases of the appendix are classified using (long) decimal numbers which begin with K35, K36, K37 or K38 and most diseases of the inner ear are classified using decimal numbers which begin with H80, H81, H82 or H83: in all cases the 'code number' is taken as a label or category.

Throughout the Health Service, there are many thousands of records like these collected every day. To make such vast quantities of data meaningful we use methods (like those described in Chapters 4 and 5) to collect them together, to present them in tables and in diagrams, and to summarise them. Returning to our present example: reports on the mean (average) length of inpatient stay for different diagnoses are commonplace. Information is also regularly displayed using graphical methods such as pie charts, bar charts, histograms, and graphs such as those included in Chapter 6.

1.2 Hip replacement by keyhole surgery

Suppose we take our data on 'inpatient stay' and from it we extract information on the mean length of hospital stay for patients undergoing a hip replacement. We wish to see whether those who have their hip replaced using keyhole surgery have, on average, a shorter stay in hospital than those whose prostheses are inserted using traditional methods.

Using the figures we presume we have collected, we see that the mean inpatient stay for patients having keyhole surgery is 9.2 days; while the mean inpatient stay for those having traditional surgery is 11.6 days.

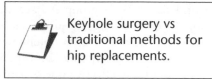

Keyhole surgery vs traditional methods for hip replacements.

Can we draw any conclusions from these figures? Can we deduce that patients who have had keyhole surgery *really do* require fewer days in hospital? – or should we be more cautious? Perhaps this is a chance result because our figures are non-standard in some way. It is possible that, among the patients we included, those who had keyhole surgery were unusually young. Or maybe in our group of patients there was a small number who underwent traditional surgery and who later developed a wound infection, leading to a prolonged inpatient stay. If we continue to collect information about more hip replacement patients, over a longer time-scale, our figures will probably support the conclusion that the two different approaches to hip replacement surgery do *not* imply different requirements for inpatient stay.

Statistics offers us ways to approach the above issues. On the one hand (as we explain in Chapter 3) it gives us ways to select a sample of patients that is truly representative so that valid deductions may be made, and it helps us to decide on the appropriate size of such a sample. On the other hand it supplies methods by which we can compare mean values and also determine how confident we are that our comparison is correct (see Chapters 9 and 10).

1.3 The effectiveness of nicotine replacement therapy

Those working in a national health service must judge carefully the efficacy of new treatment regimes and new disease prevention programmes before making decisions about their widespread adoption. Research studies are often set up to

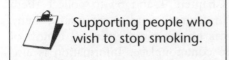
Supporting people who wish to stop smoking.

provide the evidence to support such decisions. If a new method of nicotine replacement therapy is proposed – to assist people who wish to give up smoking cigarettes – then we can adopt a 'research approach' to evaluate the new product, comparing it with an existing product.

We take two 'equivalent' groups of smokers and administer the new treatment to group A and the existing treatment to group B. After a certain time period we ascertain the proportion of people in each group who have managed to quit smoking. We expect that some people on the new treatment are still smoking, and some people on the existing treatment have stopped smoking: it is very rare indeed for a new treatment to offer 100% success, or for an old treatment to give 100% failure. (In the unlikely event of a new treatment offering 100% success rates we have little difficulty in deciding on its efficacy!) Suppose we find that 63% of group A have stopped smoking, compared with 54% of group B: do these figures justify us in concluding that the new treatment is superior to the old? This is potentially an important decision, since a mistake could mean us promoting an expensive but ineffective treatment while a cheaper but more effective one is banished.

By methods like those discussed in Chapter 3, Statistics offers us methods to ensure that the groups of people we study *will* be 'equivalent'. We also have a variety of ways to compare our results, so that we can decide whether or not they support the conclusion that one treatment *is* better than the other – or whether the differences might just be due to chance (see Chapters 9, 10 and 11).

1.4 Supporting older people in their own homes

Much of the planning for health and social care depends upon surveys of illness and the need for care in the general population. The increasing demand on residential care homes and nursing care homes leads us to examine ways in which

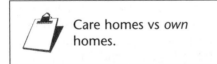
Care homes vs *own* homes.

older people can be supported in their *own* homes, for as long as possible. This involves us in estimating the extent of the extra services that will be required to realise this, that is the 'meals on wheels', the housing adaptions, the community nursing, etc. required to support older people in leading their lives independently. It is important that society gets these estimates right. If the estimates are inaccurate there are two possible outcomes: either insufficient resources will be allocated to deal with these issues, and then real needs might remain unmet – or else too much resource will be allocated in this area and then services for other members of the community will inevitably suffer.

Statistics gives us tools to help us gather information from surveys (we illustrate these in Chapter 2). It also provides techniques by which we can estimate values that are valid for a population when we have access only to some smaller sample and, essentially, it allows us to calculate the level of confidence that we have in our estimates (see Chapter 8).

1.5 Judging if a body temperature is normal

Decisions about the care and treatment of a patient are often made on the grounds that their characteristics are not within what is considered to be a normal range. Prime among these characteristics is body temperature. While there is a widely accepted rule of thumb that the normal body temperature of a healthy adult is 98.4°F (36.9°C), it has been discov-

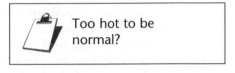

Too hot to be normal?

ered fairly recently that the average body temperature in healthy adults ranges from 97.6°F (36.4°C) to 98.8°F (37.1°C) (Shoemaker 1996). Moreover, we know that the temperature of a healthy person varies for a number of reasons: it is lower in the morning after a night's sleep, and it is higher later on in the day, after eating and after exercise. So it is important that we should be able to decide *how far* someone's temperature must rise or fall before we decide that it is no longer normal.

Once we know the distribution of measurements of body temperature, we can apply statistical methods (like those in Chapters 7 and 9) to determine how likely it is that a single patient's temperature is 'abnormal'.

1.6 Exercise and health

It is commonly believed that there is a connection between good health and exercise. Certainly if someone takes no exercise at all they are most unlikely to be healthy and, in general, people who are considered to be healthy do take regular exercise. But while we *believe* that good health and exercise are connected it is useful to be able to *demonstrate* this – perhaps to support arguments regarding 'fitness classes on prescription' or the retention of community sports facilities.

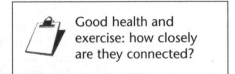

Good health and exercise: how closely are they connected?

Statistics gives us the tools to identify connections, known as correlations, between qualities like these. As we discuss in Chapter 12, it also allows us to quantify the strength of any correlation and, where appropriate, to predict values of one quality that will give us desired outcomes in the other.

1.7 The uptake of cervical smear tests

The planning and delivery of healthcare services such as cervical screening can be affected by the attitudes of the relevant population to taking up the services offered. We know that morbidity and mortality from cervical tumours can be reduced greatly by analysing cervical smears from healthy women for the purpose of early detection, but obviously this depends on women using the service. Despite the benefits, some women do not. There seem to be many reasons which *might* account for this and to improve the uptake it is useful to identify these, find if they are linked and find which are the most significant.

> Cervical screening: what factors influence the uptake?

We can collect data from large numbers of women who use the service as well as from those who do not. We collect facts covering a whole battery of variables which we think *may* have influenced their decision, knowingly or unknowingly. We might include questions on age, family history, existing level of health, marital status, number of children, frequency of visits to their GP, educational achievement, access to private transport, income etc., – this list could cover an enormous range of topics. The result is a vast amount of data concerning very many variables measured over a large number of women. From these data we would hope to extract information which we can analyse to tell us which are the important variables (or 'factors') in influencing women's behaviour. Then in the light of this knowledge, we might ultimately be able to direct resources to areas which would support the uptake of these screening tests.

The statistical methods used to disentangle the relative contributions of a multitude of variables are known as multivariate methods. They include multiple regression, the analysis of covariance and factor analysis, which we discuss briefly in Chapter 13.

1.8 Using statistics

As we see above, we meet Statistics in very many professional contexts, and we know that Statistics is used in so many ways in daily life. It is essential that we master the basic principles and processes so that we can gain for ourselves the maximum benefit from this form of information. Statistics is also misused and abused far too frequently: we need to understand the different issues involved so that we are not hoodwinked at any stage.

For Nursing and the other healthcare professions, Statistics provides a vital form of communication about patients in particular and about healthcare in general. Statistics provides essential tools in the development of evidence based practice, and health practitioners will want to have a sound grasp of them and use them with confidence.

Levels of Measurement

– using numbers to measure qualities that vary

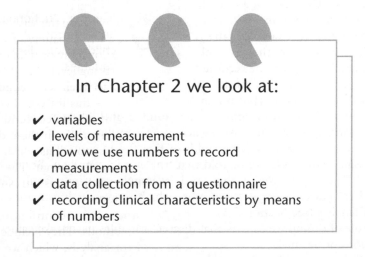

In Chapter 2 we look at:

✔ variables
✔ levels of measurement
✔ how we use numbers to record measurements
✔ data collection from a questionnaire
✔ recording clinical characteristics by means of numbers

If we need to know about supplies of dressings, we can count the boxes; if we need to know a patient's weight, we can use weighing scales; but there are also ways to measure less tangible qualities like 'level of pain' or 'level of comfort' or 'satisfaction level'. Statistical techniques are used to make sense of many different kinds of measurements so it is important that we understand what is meant by '**measurement**', what sorts of qualities can be measured and how numbers are used to record measurements.

2.1 Variables

Qualities that interest us (such as gender, age, temperature, time), that are likely to vary in different circumstances and different cases, are called **variables**. For example, in a study of hospital inpatients the length of inpatient stay will differ

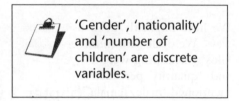

'Length of hospital stay', 'weight' and 'gender' are all variables.

from patient to patient. In this case the variable of interest is 'length of inpatient stay' and the value of the variable for each patient is counted in days. Alternatively we could be interested in the weight of each patient on admission; here the variable is 'weight of patient' and its value in each case is recorded in kilograms. If we were interested in identifying the numbers of men and women in our study the variable would be 'gender': it could have only two possible values, either 'male' or 'female'.

Discrete variables are qualities or characteristics which can be expressed only as 'separate categories' or 'separate numbers'. The value of a discrete variable is either the *name* of its category or a *number*. An example of this is 'gender', as above. Another example is 'nationality', which can be recorded as the separate values 'Scottish' or 'Ugandan' or 'Malaysian' (but no 'in-

'Gender', 'nationality' and 'number of children' are discrete variables.

between' values have any meaning!). The 'number of children in a family' is also a discrete variable: it can only take a whole number value (it is, of course, impossible to have a fraction of a living child, such as 0.4 of a girl).

In passing: why might we be told that 'the average family in Britain has 1.7 children'? The key to this is the word 'average': no *single* family can have 1.7 children, but an average is a number which represents information from a *group* of families (see Section 5.2).

As a rule of thumb we can say that discrete variables never take values which are fractions or decimals.

Continuous variables are qualities or characteristics which can be expressed as whole numbers or fractions or *any* in-between value (with no 'gaps' possible). An example of a continuous variable is 'blood glucose level', using a finger prick specimen and a blood glucose monitoring test strip. A particular value might be read as 4.8 millimoles per litre (mmol/l) for instance, and another could be 4.9

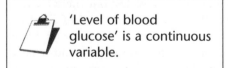

'Level of blood glucose' is a continuous variable.

mmol/l. Yet another might be 4.84 mmol/l and, depending on the accuracy of the instrument, another could be 4.863 mmol/l.

In practice we usually limit the number of decimal places we record. We 'round off' the reading for convenience, say to the first place of decimals. The first two readings above would be recorded as given, but 4.84 mmol/l would be rounded to 4.8 mmol/l and 4.863 mmol/l would be rounded to 4.9 mmol/l.

A glucose test meter used by patients is accurate to one decimal place. Thus a reading of 4.8 mmol/l indicates a true glucose level between 4.75 mmol/l and 4.84 mmol/l. If we decide to conduct the test on more expensive laboratory-based equipment then we could expect the result to be accurate to two decimal places; but even so, we would probably find the value of the approximation to *just one* place of decimals the most useful. In clinical practice blood glucose values are generally reported to only one decimal place.

Other continuous variables include weight, height, temperature and blood pressure. They can all be recorded as accurately as our equipment allows, and we usually use approximations for convenience.

2.2 Measurement

We have implicitly been using the idea of **measurement** in several different ways. We dealt with 'numbers of days' (measuring lengths of stay), 'how many kilos' (measuring weights), 'how many children' (measuring sizes of families) and 'quantity per litre' (measuring blood glucose levels). We have also mentioned 'male/female' (indicating – or measuring – gender) and 'Scottish/ Ugandan/Malaysian' (indicating – or measuring – nationality).

If such a simple classification as male or female is considered to be a form of measurement, how then is measurement defined? The widely accepted definition of measurement was proposed by Stevens (1951), it is: '. . . *the assignment of numerals to objects or events according to rules*'. Numerals are the symbols for writing numbers (1, 2, 3, etc.) and these rules are applied in a taxonomy of different **levels of measurement**, as Stevens describes.

When we measure, for example, a patient's temperature or weight or attitudes, the values recorded have properties which determine the 'level' of measurement. The four different levels of measurement in common use are **nominal**, **ordinal**, **interval** and **ratio** (their initials make the acronym **NOIR**). We now show how each level of measurement has a set of properties and we move from one level up to the next by introducing one more property.

Nominal measurement is the very lowest level of measurement (some people would say it is merely a system of classification). The only property that this level requires is that it is possible to differentiate between the classes or categories.

We have already noted that the variable 'gender' has two categories, men and women. These categories are essentially different; no similarity or difference between men and women can really be indicated just by numbers. However, for convenience and for consistency with other levels of measurement, it is useful to assign numerals as 'labels' to the categories.

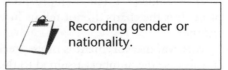

Recording gender or nationality.

Thus we can allocate '1' for 'male' and '2' for 'female': which numerals we use does not matter, so long as they are different. Similarly, for the variable 'nationality' we introduced there are three quite different categories possible; if we wish we can allocate '100' for 'Scottish', '200' for 'Ugandan' and '300' for 'Malaysian'.

Other variables whose categories/values can be 'measured' at a nominal level include a person's religion, their eye colour, their ethnic origin – and there are many more examples. Many systems of classification can be viewed as measurement at a nominal level. For example the International Classification of Diseases (ICD-10, World Health Organisation 2003) can be seen to be a measuring instrument. This classification provides a unique code number

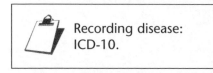

Recording disease: ICD-10.

for every diagnosis (for example: D30.2 for benign neoplasm of the ureter, J03.0 for acute streptococcal tonsillitis, N30.0 for acute cystitis) and is used throughout the world to record morbidity and mortality.

Ordinal measurement has the property of nominal measurement, but in addition the different categories can be meaningfully ranked, or ordered. It may not be possible to express the actual differences between categories using numbers, but we can still recognise a logical order between them.

For example, a patient's visual ability can be measured at an ordinal level as being 'effectively blind', 'partial vision' or 'full vision'. Here the variable 'visual ability' takes three possible values: the categories 'effectively

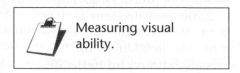

Measuring visual ability.

blind', 'partial vision' and 'full vision'. At this level we cannot express the actual difference between the categories by numbers, but we *can* appreciate a logical order here: 'effectively blind' is *less than* 'partial vision' and 'full vision' is *more than* 'partial vision'. To allocate numbers to such ranked categories it is usual to assign the lowest number to the lowest-ranked category and the highest to the highest-ranked category. It is important that numbers are assigned to categories in the same relative order as in the ranking. Thus for 'visual ability' we could assign 'effectively blind' = 1, 'partial vision' = 2 and 'full vision' = 3.

Other examples of variables whose values/categories can be measured at an ordinal level include 'nursing grade', where the categories are the D, E, F, G, H and I grades. The popular music industry also uses an ordinal system of measurement when it publishes the weekly chart successes. We know that the week's 'Number 1 Hit' is more popular than the record in second or third place, but the charts do not tell us how much more popular one single is than another.

Interval measurement is more precise than the two levels already described. In this case the numbers assigned to the values/categories being measured truly reflect these values in a *quantitative* way. Interval measurement has the properties of ordinal measurement, but, in addition, the differences between the categories are assumed to be quantitatively equal.

In this situation we assign numbers to values as if they lie on a scale, like the degrees marked on the glass of a thermometer. As is obvious from this example, the number 'zero' has no intrinsic meaning in interval measure: it is the *difference* between two readings that matters. When reading temperatures, the *difference* between 10°C and 11°C is exactly the same as the *difference*

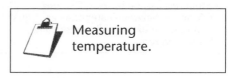

Measuring temperature.

between 20°C and 21°C, that is, one degree Celcius. The zero on the Celcius scale is (arbitrarily) located at the temperature where water freezes (but note – this is *not* the temperature where there is a complete absence of heat). The consequence of this is that when a temperature rises from 10°C to 20°C, we can*not* say that it has become 'twice as hot'.

Many qualities of interest to nursing and to healthcare research are measured at an interval level. Apart from temperature, the time of day (but not the duration of time itself) is also measured at this level: hours on a clock indicate equal time intervals, but '4 o'clock' does not measure 'twice as much time' as '2 o'clock'. In addition, attitude scales such as the Lickert Scale and some scaled measures of patient satisfaction use measurement at an interval level.

Ratio measurement is the highest and most precise level of measurement. Measurements at this level have all the properties of interval measurement and in addition the 'zero measure' is fixed. 'Zero' has an intrinsic meaning with regard to the variable concerned; there is an absolute zero as the lowest possible measure and there can be no negative values. At this level, the numbers assigned by the measurements can be manipulated in exactly the same way as in school arithmetic; they can be added, subtracted, multiplied and divided.

Qualities which can be measured at this level include height, volume, weight, family size, etc. They are commonly encountered in the physical environment and are important in clinical practice – the concept 'zero' has a real meaning. In

Measuring height, weight, family size.

addition, duration of time is also measured at ratio level: a period of one minute (from a 'time zero' perhaps set by a stop-watch) *is* twice as long as a period of thirty seconds, and 'zero duration' *does* have real meaning.

The properties of measurements which determine which level is being used are summarised in Table 2.1.

In Table 2.2 we summarise which type of measurement can be applied to discrete variables and which to continuous variables. In general, whenever a particular level *can* be applied then, if it is thought appropriate, any lower level measurement *may* be applied.

Table 2.1 The properties of measurements at different levels

	Levels of measurement			
Property	*Nominal*	*Ordinal*	*Interval*	*Ratio*
Has different categories	✔	✔	✔	✔
Categories can be ranked		✔	✔	✔
Differences between categories are equal and can be expressed numerically			✔	✔
Has a fixed zero				✔

Table 2.2 The levels of measurement which can be applied to the different types of variables, with examples

In Row A we have the different types of variables and in Row B we show the possible levels of measurement which can be applied to them.

Here are examples of variables which can be measured at the levels shown:

	Discrete (*names*)	Discrete (*numbers*)	Continuous
Nominal	nationality	bus numbers	
Ordinal	grades of mobility (poor/fair/good)	class of travel (1st, 2nd, 3rd . . .)	
Interval		IQ scores	temperature
Ratio		family size	weight

2.3 Collecting data, a practical example

When we want information about certain qualities of interest, then we collect **data** (noting that this is a 'plural' word) about them, and the level of measurement we apply to the values, or categories, affects the organisation and the analysis we can subsequently use. Data recorded at a higher level of measurement are more precise so more powerful methods of statistical analysis can be used on them. In general it is desirable to collect research data at high levels of measurement.

We now look at a practical example of how data can be collected. Table 2.3 is a questionnaire with seven questions, designed to be distributed to hospital nursing staff. The intention is to collect information regarding seven variables:

Table 2.3 A questionnaire for hospital based nursing staff

1. Tick a box to indicate your gender   Male ☐ 1
                                                   Female ☐ 2

2. What is your age in years?   Years ☐☐

3. At what grade of nurse are you employed?
Tick appropriate box . . .

                     4   5   6
                     D☐   E☐   F☐
                     7   8   9
                     G☐   H☐   I☐

4. Are you employed full-time or part-time?
Tick appropriate box . . .   Part-time ☐ 1
                                               Full-time ☐ 2

5. Please describe your clinical area of work.
e.g. Acute medical ward/Out-patient dept . . . . ☐

6. On the line below please ring a number to show how
satisfied you are with the quality of care that is provided to
patients in your ward or department

     1   2   3   4   5   6   7   8   9   10
     completely   completely
     dissatisfied   satisfied

7. If you are less than completely satisfied please explain why.   ☐
. . . .
. . . .

gender, age, grade, full-time or part-time employment, area of work, level of satisfaction with the quality of care provided and any reasons for being less than satisfied with that care. The answers to these questions provide examples of categories/values at all the different levels of measurement discussed, i.e. nominal, ordinal, interval and ratio. In addition, the final question asks for data which are not obviously susceptible to 'measurement'. However, we shall show that these data also can be dealt with quantitatively.

Sometimes there is no choice about the level at which data values are measured. This is true for *Question 1*, where the variable 'gender' has just two categories and the nominal level of measurement is the only one possible. This variable is also discrete, so the numerals we shall use to identify and record the categories are 'male = 1' and 'female = 2'.

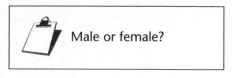

Male or female?

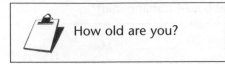

How old are you?

Question 2 asks for the respondent's age in (completed) years. The variable 'age' is continuous and its values *could* contain fractions or decimals, but here the question is phrased so that individual ages are rounded down to the nearest whole number of years, so we have a discrete variable. The numerals recorded are the nurses' ages at last birthday, and zero *would* have an intrinsic meaning: this variable is measured at ratio level.

Question 2 is a situation where we can *choose* the level at which data values are measured. As a general rule we might aim for the *highest* level of measurement, but this can have costs. When we measure the values at ratio level we get high precision results, but we might lose out if some people refused to complete the questionnaire since they object to revealing their exact age. This problem can be resolved by lowering the level of measurement we will accept.

Suppose that Question 2 were posed as in Table 2.4, asking for ages to be indicated within roughly ten-year bands. Since no *exact* ages need be revealed, we would hope that this might increase the numbers of people completing the questionnaire, but we have reduced the level of measurement to ordinal. We would know that all the people in the 21–30 years category are younger than all those in the 31–40 years category, but we could not know by how many years: this loss of precision may or may not be important.

We see that once we have collected data then the level of measurement *can be reduced* but the opposite is not true; the level of measurement *can never be increased* once the data have been collected. We must bear this in mind when designing research and making proposals for data collection and analysis. If data from particular variables are considered vital, then we may prefer to go for as precise a level of measurement as possible and deal with the issues of possible non-response by other methods. These methods might include increasing the explanations given with the questionnaires and/or giving additional assurances about confidentiality to encourage co-operation.

Table 2.4   Measuring age at an ordinal level

2. Please tick a box to indicate which age group you belong.

21 to 30 years	☐	1
31 to 40 years	☐	2
41 to 50 years	☐	3
51 to 60 years	☐	4
61 years or over	☐	5

Question 3 on the questionnaire asks for nursing grade from D to I: this variable is being measured at ordinal level. In the nursing hierarchy we know that D is lower than E, and E is lower than F, etc., but the actual differences between the grades cannot be described by numbers. The numbers indicated beside the boxes are used rather like labels and arranged in the 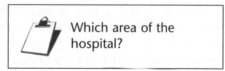 same relative order as the ranking. That is, the lowest grade 'D' is given the lowest number '4', then the numbers increase grade by grade until the highest grade 'I' gets the highest number '9'.

For *Question 4* the variable 'full-time or part-time employment' has the two categories 'full-time' and 'part-time'. These are here measured at an ordinal level, so as part-time staff work fewer hours than full-time staff the allocations are '1' for 'part-time' and '2' for 'full-time'. While we choose to accept this level of measurement as adequate, in other circumstances we might 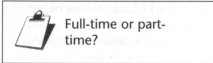 require the values of this variable to be given in the exact number of hours and minutes worked each week: this would raise the level of measurement to ratio.

Question 5 asks about the area of work of each respondent and since the information yields unordered categories it is obviously measured at a nominal level. Especially in a large hospital, the responses will be very varied, so generally we wait until all the data are collected before classifying answers or allocating numerals. Once all the questionnaires have been returned we group the responses into categories; the procedure for this classification must be clearly defined. Then we label each category with a numeral and, as before, the actual numerals used are irrelevant as long as they are all different. We might propose the following: 1 = Acute Medical, 2 = Acute Surgical, 3 = Orthopaedics, 4 = Gynaecology, 5 = ENT, 6 = OPD, 7 = A&E, 8 = other and 9 = 'response missing'. In **coding schemes** like this it is always sensible to include extra categories for 'other' and 'response missing', which are used for replies which do not fit into the main categories or where a respondent has omitted to answer the question.

In *Question 6* we ask that 'level of satisfaction' be shown by ringing a number on an **equal appearing interval scale**. This scale has apparently equal intervals marked between 1 and 10 along a straight line (obviously there is no 'real' meaning to the number zero). These data fulfil the requirements for measurement at an interval level.

Generally, 'satisfaction' can also be measured at nominal and ordinal levels, but this type of scale is a very popular way of measuring the intensity of personal feelings and attitudes.

In *Question 7* we ask for subjective opinions. In themselves these are incapable of measurement, but there *is* a way to deal with them in a numerical framework. The procedure involves scrutinising a sample of responses and developing a set of categories which can best accommodate the comments. For example we may find that responses frequently refer to issues of management, staffing levels, staff training and available equipment/facilities. We group all the comments from the nurses into these categories, including importantly 'other', 'not applicable' and 'missing'. In this way the subjective responses are converted into categories which can be measured at a nominal level; the labels used could be 1 = management, 2 = staffing levels, 3 = staff training, 4 = available equipment/facilities, 5 = other, 6 = N/A, 7 = 'response missing'.

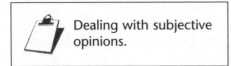
Dealing with subjective opinions.

In dealing with classifications for subjective information we can apply different approaches of different complexity; the one just described is fairly simple. We could alternatively decide to look within the comments for attitudes towards management and then classify these as positive, neutral or negative. This would increase the level of precision as the variable could be measured at an ordinal level. However, we should be very careful here: while it is certainly possible to carry out such a manipulation it is not always wise practice. If a researcher needs to find out about nurses' views of management it is far preferable to ask them directly. Interpreting comments inevitably introduces the possibility of bias and lays any findings open to criticism.

2.4 Tabulating data

Having dealt in detail with the measurement of the variables used in the questionnaire, we show in Table 2.5 the actual data collected from a sample of 120 nurses.

Each respondent's answers contribute one row of numerical data and there are 60 rows in each rectangle. The columns have headings to represent the questions. The first column in each rectangle contains a personal identifier (ID No.) between 000 and 119. The meanings of the numbers in the remaining columns are shown in Table 2.6. Such a **coding key** for any data set should always be recorded.

We now look at the data set presented in Table 2.5: can we begin to develop a picture of its meaning 'in our mind's eye'? Most people give up rapidly on this – they conclude that the table is just a meaningless jumble of numbers! To begin to make sense of it we must apply some methods to organise it and to

Table 2.5 Sample data obtained from questionnaire (no. of respondents = 120)

ID No.	Sex	Age	Grade	PT-FT	Area	Satis	Explain
00	1	30	6	2	2	5	5
01	1	35	4	2	5	9	2
02	1	41	7	2	2	5	1
03	2	42	6	1	1	6	2
04	2	34	5	2	4	3	2
05	2	39	4	2	1	5	2
06	1	47	4	2	1	5	3
07	2	55	4	2	2	5	1
08	1	30	4	2	2	4	2
09	1	33	5	2	3	6	3
10	2	25	6	1	3	8	2
11	2	27	7	1	1	5	1
12	2	33	6	2	2	5	1
13	1	54	9	1	3	7	3
14	2	37	7	2	1	5	4
15	2	41	5	2	2	9	1
16	2	39	5	2	6	6	5
17	2	33	6	1	1	6	5
18	1	42	4	1	5	1	6
19	2	34	7	2	1	6	5
20	2	21	6	2	4	10	6
21	2	42	5	2	2	1	2
22	1	26	4	2	1	3	4
23	1	36	7	2	4	4	4
24	2	46	8	1	2	4	4
25	2	51	9	1	4	9	2
26	2	33	8	2	2	5	4
27	2	56	7	2	6	4	1
28	1	27	5	1	6	5	1
29	2	49	7	2	1	2	2
30	2	32	5	2	4	5	2
31	2	42	9	2	2	3	2
32	2	38	8	2	5	6	1
60	2	31	7	2	6	4	2
61	2	28	8	2	2	7	1
62	1	54	5	2	2	7	1
63	2	27	4	2	1	5	2
64	2	49	7	2	2	6	2
65	2	30	5	1	1	4	2
66	1	26	7	2	1	6	1
67	2	26	5	1	4	4	3
68	2	39	9	2	2	6	5
69	2	28	8	2	2	7	5
70	2	36	7	2	3	5	1
71	1	37	4	1	4	6	1
72	2	32	7	2	7	10	6
73	1	32	6	1	4	8	3
74	2	40	4	1	4	7	2
75	1	33	8	1	2	4	2
76	1	39	4	2	2	8	3
77	2	21	5	2	4	6	1
78	2	27	4	2	3	4	2
79	2	24	5	1	3	5	1
80	2	50	8	2	1	6	1
81	1	30	4	2	2	8	3
82	1	22	7	2	5	3	2
83	2	31	5	2	7	3	4
84	2	34	6	2	2	2	4
85	2	35	7	1	1	2	2
86	2	44	6	1	5	4	2
87	2	58	4	2	1	2	2
88	1	40	8	2	5	10	6
89	1	31	7	2	1	5	3
90	2	40	4	2	4	6	3
91	1	49	4	2	4	7	2
92	2	56	6	1	7	7	2

Table 2.5 *continued*

ID No.	Sex	Age	Grade	PT-FT	Area	Satis	Explain
33	2	32	5	2	2	7	3
34	1	28	7	2	7	6	2
35	1	52	6	1	2	8	1
36	2	41	4	2	3	4	4
37	2	37	4	2	1	4	1
38	2	32	4	2	5	6	2
39	2	38	4	2	1	5	2
40	2	43	7	1	7	9	1
41	2	52	5	2	1	6	4
42	2	51	5	2	2	6	2
43	1	23	5	2	7	8	2
44	2	25	6	1	1	9	1
45	1	34	9	2	5	8	2
46	1	25	5	2	5	3	5
47	1	29	8	2	2	3	2
48	2	35	8	2	3	2	2
49	1	27	4	2	3	7	1
50	2	39	5	1	3	7	2
51	2	46	4	2	7	6	3
52	2	44	4	2	1	6	1
53	1	42	4	2	2	2	3
54	2	57	4	2	4	6	1
55	2	28	4	2	3	6	2
56	2	51	6	2	4	2	1
57	1	26	6	2	5	7	3
58	2	48	4	2	4	5	2
59	2	50	6	2	1	2	1
93	2	53	6	1	6	5	3
94	1	37	7	2	1	3	3
95	2	37	4	1	2	3	2
96	2	44	7	2	4	4	5
97	2	46	4	2	1	1	1
98	2	26	5	1	1	7	2
99	2	56	6	2	3	4	5
100	1	28	4	1	2	4	4
101	1	49	6	1	4	6	2
102	1	27	6	2	5	3	3
103	1	31	5	1	3	4	5
104	2	37	6	1	1	5	1
105	1	27	6	1	2	9	2
106	2	30	4	1	2	5	4
107	1	38	6	1	3	7	3
108	2	33	6	2	4	6	5
109	2	41	6	2	6	3	2
110	1	36	5	1	4	1	3
111	1	25	4	1	3	2	1
112	2	24	4	1	3	4	5
113	2	28	6	2	2	4	5
114	1	27	4	2	1	5	2
115	2	32	5	1	1	6	3
116	2	35	6	2	5	4	1
117	1	44	5	1	2	7	1
118	1	31	5	2	2	5	1
119	2	29	4	2	1	3	4

Table 2.6 Coding key for data shown in Table 2.5

Question No.	Column heading	Variable	Values
1	Sex	Gender	1 = Male 2 = Female
2	Age	Age in years	Number of years
3	Grade	Nursing grade	4 = D 5 = E 6 = F 7 = G 8 = H 9 = I
4	PT-FT	Employed PT or FT	1 = Part-time 2 = Full-time
5	Area	Clinical area	1 = Acute Medical 2 = Acute Surgical 3 = Orthopaedics 4 = Gynaecology 5 = ENT 6 = OPD 7 = A&E 8 = Other 9 = Missing
6	Satis	Satisfaction with level of care	(Scale value 1 to 10) 1 = Completely dissatisfied 10 = Completely satisfied
7	Explain	Explanation for lack of satisfaction	1 = Management 2 = Staffing levels 3 = Staff training 4 = Available equipment/ facilities 5 = Other 6 = n/a 7 = Missing

summarise it: for this we need the tools of 'descriptive statistics', which we begin to introduce in Chapter 4.

2.5 Some measurements in healthcare

In this section we look at how the principles discussed above can be applied to data collected in certain clinical practice. We discuss the meaning of the 'scores' which some clinical investigations produce, and investigate some of their underlying assumptions.

For a variety of reasons it can be very appealing and very convenient to be able to 'sum up' a patient's characteristics using numbers. If a patient is allocated a single number which is the value of a particular variable, then that can support administrative and clinical management decisions. If the assigned number has been determined by an apparently tested 'scientific' scale and the measurements are at an interval or even ratio level, then so much the better. However, the use of a single overall score, purporting to amalgamate meaningfully the measures of several different variables, is an exercise which can have many pitfalls. These scores are widely used, but we should be aware that they can bring their own problems with them.

There are very many different summary scales available to healthcare professionals. We can imagine a situation where a patient arrives with a Waterlow pressure sore risk score of 20, a Barthel functional ability index score of 64, a Mini mental state score of 5, a caregiver burden inventory score of 83 and a CAS (constipation assessment scale) score of 17. We should be fairly confident that we knew a great deal about

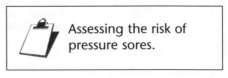

Many scales can be applied to the same patient!

their condition before we even set eyes on them! As examples of these scoring systems (and their pros and cons) we next take closer, critical looks at the Waterlow pressure sore risk Scale (Waterlow 1985) and the Barthel Index of functional ability (Mahoney & Barthel 1965).

The Waterlow Scale provides a score between 1 and 65 to represent the risk of a patient developing a pressure sore. The greater the score then the greater the likelihood of pressure sores developing. To determine the score a clinician assesses fifteen variables: seven patient attributes and eight special risk factors (shown in Table 2.7). These fifteen separate numbers are added together to produce the overall score.

Assessing the risk of pressure sores.

The Barthel Index provides a score between zero and 100 which reflects a person's functional ability: a high degree of functional ability gets a high score and as functional ability decreases so the score gets lower. A person's ability at ten different daily activities is scored between zero and 15 (see Table 2.8); the final score is obtained by adding these ten numbers.

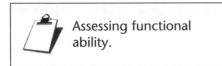

Assessing functional ability.

Looking at both the Waterlow Scale and the Barthel Index we should be aware that whenever we use a single number to 'sum up' a group of characteristics, each of which has been allocated a separate score, then we are making some *important* assumptions.

The first assumption is that the overall scale is **uni-dimensional** – it must be concerned with measuring a single overall variable. In the case of the Waterlow Scale that variable is 'risk of pressure sores'; in the case of the Barthel Index it is 'functional ability'.

Table 2.7   The Waterlow pressure sore risk calculator

Attribute	
Sex	1 = male 2 = female
Age	1 = 14–49 2 = 50–64 3 = 65–74 4 = 75–80 5 = >81
Build weight for height	0 = average 1 = above average 2 = obese 3 = below average
Appetite	0 = average 1 = poor 2 = naso-gastric (NG) tube 2 = fluids only 3 = nothing by mouth anorexic
Continence	0 = complete (urine and stool) 0 = catheterised and continent faeces 1 = occasionally incontinent 2 = catheterised and incontinent faeces 3 = doubly incontinent
Mobility	0 = fully 1 = restless or fidgety 2 = apathetic 3 = restricted 4 = inert or in traction 5 = chair-bound
Skin type visual appearance in risk areas	0 = healthy 1 = tissue paper 1 = dry 1 = oedematous 1 = clammy 2 = discoloured 3 = broken spot
Special risk factors	
Terminal cachexia	8
Cardiac failure	5
Peripheral vascular disease	5
Anaemia	2
Smoking	1
Neurological deficit	4 = moderate 5 = moderate-to-sever 6 = severe
Major surgery or trauma	5 = orthopaedic below waist or spinal 5 = on table >2 hours
Medication	4 = steroids, cytotoxic agents, high dose anti-inflammatory agents

Table 2.8   The Barthel Index

Activity	Scoring
Feeding	0 = unable 5 = needs help cutting, spreading butter, etc., or requires modified diet 10 = independent
Bathing	0 = dependent 5 = independent (or in shower)
Grooming	0 = needs to help with personal care 5 = independent face/hair/teeth/shaving (implements provided)
Dressing	0 = dependent 5 = needs help but can do about half unaided 10 = independent (including buttons, zips, laces, etc.)
Bowels	0 = incontinent (or needs to be given enemas) 5 = occasional accident 10 = continent
Bladder	0 = incontinent, or catheterised and unable to manage alone 5 = occasional accident 10 = continent
Toilet use	0 = dependent 5 = needs some help, but can do something alone 10 = independent (on and off, dressing, wiping)
Transfers (bed to chair and back)	5 = unable, no sitting balance 5 = major help (one or two people, physical), can sit 10 = minor help (verbal or physical) 15 = independent
Mobility (on level surfaces)	0 = immobile or <50 yards 5 = wheelchair independent, including corners, >50 yards 10 = walks with help of one person (verbal or physical) >50 yards 15 = independent (but may use any aid; for example, stick) >50 yards
Stairs	0 = unable 5 = needs help (verbal, physical, carrying aid) 10 = independent

Mahoney FI, Barthel D. 'Functional Evaluation: The Barthel Index.' Maryland State Med Journal 1965; 14: 56–61. Used with permission

The second assumption is that the overall scale indicates the overall risk in a **logically increasing** fashion. Thus the case in reality where the overall risk is known to be least must be allocated the lowest score. The real-life case that is known to have the highest overall risk must have the highest overall score. And where one overall risk is actually greater than another, the score of the first must be greater than the second. Since we assume that all the scores are equally spaced, we see that we are here dealing with an interval level of measurement overall.

In view of what we know about levels of measurement, we now look critically at the Waterlow Scale. In Table 2.7 we see the fifteen different contributory variables whose values contribute to the overall score. Each of these variables is allocated a number which represents the amount of risk it contributes to the overall likelihood of the patient developing a pressure sore.

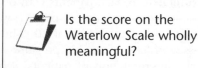

Is the score on the Waterlow Scale wholly meaningful?

The first variable appears to be 'gender', which could be measured only at a nominal level. However the variable is actually 'the contribution made by gender to overall risk'. Thus the numbers allocated, 1 = male and 2 = female, do *not just* represent the categories of male or female, they in fact represent the relative contributions of the genders to the overall risk. As 2 is greater than 1, they indicate that a woman is more likely to develop pressure sores than a man. But just as in the example of temperatures (see Section 2.2) we do not assume that a woman is *twice* as likely to develop pressure sores as a man. On this scale zero does not have any real meaning; it is an interval level of measurement being applied.

The second variable appears to be 'age', which could be measured at a ratio level, or – since here the ages are grouped – at an ordinal level of measurement. But in fact the variable is actually 'the contribution made by age to overall risk'. The numbers from 1 to 5 are not used merely as labels, or to indicate order, but they represent interval levels of the measurement of this risk. Zero on this scale has no 'real' meaning, and it does *not* follow from ' "1" = 14–49' and ' "3" = 65–74' that a person aged 70 is three times more likely to develop pressure sores than someone aged 15.

The third variable is 'the contribution made by physical build to the risk of developing pressure sores'. This can only be measured at an ordinal level, but, but since the increasing risks are allocated scores from 0 to 3 we see that an interval level of measurement is implied. However, there is more here! The score of zero exists and it corresponds to the 'real' case that a person of average build has zero risk (from their build) of developing pressure sores. Thus we here have a ratio level of measurement.

We shall not consider every one of the contributory variables in this detail, but we have done enough to show the apparent lack of consistency. We now consider the *overall* risk score obtained by adding together the fifteen contributory scores. This figure appears to be on an interval scale (with no meaningful zero). However, doubtful results arise: the overall risk score of a woman smoker aged 20 who is slightly below average weight comes out the same as that of a 64 year old doubly incontinent man of average weight. Common sense tells us that this is unlikely to be true! The scale is not operating at an interval level of measurement, nor is it increasing in a logical fashion. In addition, we cannot guarantee that this scale is uni-dimensional! The precursors of pressure sores are not fully understood: we have no guarantee that we have considered *all* the contributing risks or even only those that are relevant, nor can we be sure that the scores are combined in appropriate proportion.

Where does this uncertainty leave nurses who use the Waterlow Scale in practice? We have shown that the overall score does not use an interval level of measurement. In fact, patients with obviously different overall risks can achieve the same scores and a score of 40 (say) might in reality indicate only a *slightly* increased risk over a score of 20. The Waterlow Scale certainly serves to raise the issue of 'consistency' in pressure sore risk assessment, but, to be meaningful, the interpretation of patients' scores requires the judicious use of much professional knowledge and experience.

Finally, we can make similar comments about the Barthel Index; it too runs into difficulties in the way that measurements are used. The contributory variables are each measured at an ordinal level naturally, but then scores at an interval level are applied to the ordinally defined categories. Thus we face the same problems as with the Waterlow Scale. The scores of the categories which contribute to functional ability are assumed to contribute proportionally to the overall score, but 'needing assistance to dress' has the same score as 'occasional accidental incontinence' – which goes against common sense. Because the overall score has an ostensibly meaningful zero and ranges from 0 to 100, we might gain the impression that it has a ratio level of measurement. However, unless a patient is unconscious, the idea of *no* functional ability is an unreal extreme. Neither can we claim that a score of 50 would represent 'half of the functional ability' of someone with a score of 100. The combination of scores also raises issues about uni-dimensionality and about the logical progression of the scores.

Is the score from the Barthel Index completely logical?

Like the Waterlow Scale, the Barthel Index fails to provide a scale where the scores are consistent with their level of measurement, or, indeed, with the reality they supposedly represent. The rules outlined by Stevens (1951) have been infringed in both cases and so the overall scores from both must be viewed with caution – or even scepticism. The use of these scales cannot replace clinical judgement.

Populations and Samples
3

– using sampling techniques to generate data

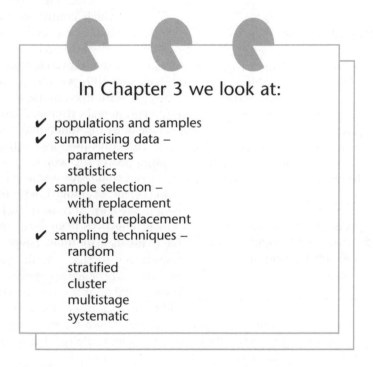

In Chapter 3 we look at:

✔ populations and samples
✔ summarising data –
    parameters
    statistics
✔ sample selection –
    with replacement
    without replacement
✔ sampling techniques –
    random
    stratified
    cluster
    multistage
    systematic

In any professional context we wish our planning and our decision making to have a firm basis, supported by useful **information** which has been appropriately analysed. We get such information by organising and summarising our original (raw) **data**, as we shall show in following chapters, but before we do this we must decide *how do we obtain the data*? There are many possible methods we can choose, among them questionnaires (such as Table 2.3) or direct measurements (for heights, weights, blood pressures, etc.) or informed observation (as for the Barthel Index or Waterlow Scale, see Section 2.5).

But before we apply any of these methods, there is another level of decision to be made here: *who (or what) do we obtain the data from?* Ideally, we might like to collect data from *everyone* or *everything* involved, but very often this is impossible or impractical and we have to 'make do' with a **sample**. The choice of our sample is crucial. In seeking nurses' opinions on a general matter we would not consider it sensible to canvas opinion *only* from a sample of nurses in Grade G or above. In measuring overall growth rates of infants we would not regard the results as valid if they were based *only* on a sample of those born prematurely. In judging the improved mobility claimed by a new design of crutches, could our sample sensibly be restricted to men? or to those in a particular local NHS area under 50 years old? or to the people booked into our Out-patients Clinic this week? To avoid potentially disastrous consequences, it is important that we choose our samples wisely, understanding the nature of sampling.

3.1 Populations

In a survey or a research endeavour we generally have an idea of the 'the whole' set of people or events or objects about which we wish to make statements. This 'whole set' is called the **population** we are dealing with; the term means 'everyone, or everything, that we are interested in'. This definition of 'population' is rather different from the standard 'all the people in a particular city or country' and it depends upon the purpose of our research. In defining a population we also specify the individual units (called **sampling units**) that together make up the population; any of these may be included in a sample taken from the population. The sampling units may be people or events or objects, and it may – or may not – be theoretically possible to list them all. For example, if the population is that of all qualified midwives whose names appear on the professional register on 1st January 2006, then clearly a (long) list exists.

> Can we list all qualified midwives? Could we list all sets of weighing scales?

But if the population consists of all the sets of scales used for weighing infants in Great Britain during the year 2006, then it is unfeasible (probably impossible) to consider listing them all.

Human populations are often used for studies. An example is 'All people, aged over 70, admitted to the Accident and Emergency Department of any NHS hospital in England during 2006'. However, there are many occasions when the definition of the human population is more complex than this, such as when a very precise pathology must be specified in clinical trials testing a new treatment.

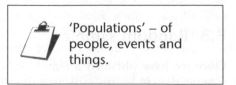

> 'Populations' – of people, events and things.

Non-human populations are just as common and, very often, it is *events* that are of interest. A hospital management might be concerned about the number of inpatients having accidents on the wards. To explore the causes for these accidents in a given period, the population of the events would be defined in as much detail as required. Other examples of possible populations of events are 'All road traffic accidents in a particular area', 'All episodes of staff absence through sickness', 'All needle stick injuries' and 'All instances of patient self-discharge from specific wards' – all defined in a given time-frame.

Sometimes *objects* are the subject of research. Quality control studies regularly focus on populations of objects. For example, if we wish to make a statement about the quality of a consignment of disposable syringes delivered to a hospital, then we can take the whole consignment as a population and every syringe in the consignment is a sampling unit in that population.

When we are able to provide figures which 'sum up' a *whole population* (like *mean, median* or *variance* which we introduce in Chapter 5), then these figures are called **parameters** ('parameters refer to populations'). Thus the average age of a population, say the average age of all non-clinical staff working in National Health Trusts in a specified region, is a parameter. The only way to obtain the value of a parameter *directly* is by a **census**, where *everyone* is dealt with individually.

3.2 Samples

Although we are generally interested in gaining information about a whole population, it is usually impractical (if not impossible) to obtain data from *every* unit in the population, because of the scale of investigation that would be required. So we use procedures to identify and select a sub-set of the population, called a **sample**, and we obtain data from the units in the sample. If the sample is obtained 'properly' and is genuinely representative of the population then there are ways in which we can use the *sample data* to give us an estimate for the corresponding figures in the *population*.

When data from a sample are summarised (to give, for example, *mean, median* or *variance* – see Chapter 5), the figures we get are called **statistics** ('statistics refer to samples'). This *second meaning* of the word 'statistics' is a special one, and quite separate from the meaning we met in Chapter 1 (where 'Statistics' is the whole subject area of collecting, organising and manipulating data). Rather than use a census to find the population parameter 'the average age of all non-clinical staff working in National Health Trusts in a specified region', we take a *sample* of the population and we calculate the *sample statistic* by finding the average age of that set of people.

3.3 Random samples

Once we have obtained a sample from a population, we want to be able to assume that it is 'truly representative' of the population in every way that

matters; only then can we be justified in using our 'statistics' to provide estimates for the 'parameters'. Thus in selecting individual sampling units from a
population, we want to be sure that our **sampling procedures** deliver a **representative sample**.

One such sampling procedure is called **simple random sampling**. In daily
life we might use the word 'random' to mean 'haphazard' or 'irregular', but
here it has a different, very specific meaning. A random sample minimises bias
by ensuring that every unit in the population has an *equal* and *independent*
chance of being selected for the sample, and so every possible sample – of a
given size – stands an equal chance of being selected in any study. There is no
better way to obtain a 'representative' sample than by using simple random
sampling. However, we can never *guarantee* that any one sample by itself is
truly representative; often we take multiple samples.

To obtain a simple random sample we need a complete list of all the units
(people, events or objects) in the population we are studying; this list is called
the **sampling frame**. The list can be organised in many different ways – for
instance alphabetically, numerically, or by age, or height, or time – but it must
be totally inclusive (no omissions) and contain no duplicates or spurious items.

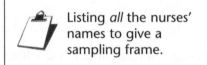
Listing *all* the nurses'
names to give a
sampling frame.

As an example we consider the alphabetical list of the population of the
thousand qualified nurses working in
a district general hospital. Every
nurse's name must be on the list, or
else they would have *no chance* at all of
being selected in the sample. If a
nurse's name appears twice on the list (erroneously) then, compared with their
colleagues, they would have a *double chance* of being selected in the sample. If
this list contains spurious names, such as those of retired nurses or those who
have moved to other hospitals, then they do not fall within the definition of our
population and so any sample is likely to be *contaminated* with units from a
different population. It is not always easy to construct an exact sampling frame
for human (or non-human) populations.

As we mentioned above, in a simple random sample *every* sampling unit has
an *equal* chance of being selected. In theory, this means that all the units in the
population should have an equal chance of being selected every time a selection
is made. This can only happen when we select every time from the *whole* population, but this allows the possibility of any one unit being selected more than
once. Especially when dealing with objects this can be quite acceptable: a unit
having been selected is 'returned to the population' where it is available to be
selected again, thus occurring more than once in the sample. This procedure is
known as **sampling with replacement**. However, in studies of human populations we usually want separate people in our samples and do not want the possibility of 'repeated sampling units'. In this case we apply **sampling without
replacement** and once a name is selected we do *not* 'return it to the population'. As long as the population is large enough, this is regarded as acceptable

practice: the difference between the chance of 'one in 1000' (when sampling with replacement) and 'one in 999' or 'one in 998' (when sampling without replacement) is *very small indeed*.

When we have established a sampling frame, the easiest way for us to identify a simple random sample is by 'labelling' every unit in the list using a set of consecutive numbers. The list of our population of nurses can be labelled with the numbers from '000' to '999' and the sample is obtained using these. How do we make a random selection from this list? There are many different ways, but we can illustrate the key idea by calling to mind the rotating drum containing numbered balls, which gives the winning numbers in the Lottery, or in tombola. We *could* have a thousand similar balls each labelled with a number from '000' to '999' and, when any one ball is released from the drum, the correspondingly numbered unit is included in our sample; this method ensures that every unit has the same chance of being chosen. However, it is unfeasible to consider this set-up with a thousand balls altogether, so we suppose we have *ten* balls, each labelled with one of the digits from '0' to '9'. Then we obtain a *random digit* by turning the drum, releasing a ball, recording the digit and returning the ball to the drum (this is *sampling with replacement*); and each sample of three random digits gives us one of the numbers between '000' and '999'. By repeating this as many times as needed we select a random sample of our population of nurses.

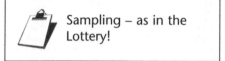

Sampling – as in the Lottery!

However, we see that even this second method is time-consuming and impractical; in practice we make a random selection using **random numbers**. There are computer packages that will produce random numbers on command but for small scale situations we can use digits from a **Random Number Table**, such as in Appendix 5(a). Here we see some columns of random numbers: they are lists of numbers which we can imagine have been obtained by repeated use of a lottery-type drum of balls numbered from '0' to '9'. (In fact they have been produced using a computer program. By definition, it is *theoretically impossible* to predict the next random number in any list – or it would not be 'random'; but in practice these lists of numbers produced by a computer pass most of the tests for being 'random'. Technically these lists contain 'pseudo-random numbers'.)

To show how a Random Number Table can be used, we look at the relatively small section shown in Table 3.1. The digits are grouped in threes for the sake of our example, but the printed grouping is arbitrary and may always be rearranged (into pairs or fours, for example). If we wish to select a sample of twenty-five nurses at random from our sampling frame of one thousand names, we need a total of twenty-five

Listing *just some* nurses' names to form a random sample.

Table 3.1   A section from a table of random numbers

510	316	956	560	033*	799	643	257
816	628	670	703	374*	741	649	842
048	288	886	867	772	255*	576	078
229	680	048	481*	142*	578	506	258
286	405	112	128*	829	312*	236*	987
140	770	350	503	387*	947	625	545
723	595	359	595	501	652	643	812
648	319	840	408*	786	640	343*	021
388	392	747	479*	945	227*	974	795
175	057	183	831	167*	921	401	963
819	634	940	403*	305*	565	207	958
767	739	891	918	962	704	497	216
052	862	110*	102*	278*	332*	948	867
532	882	416*	163*	396*	749	653	822
700	737	095*	952	261*	994	619	084

Generated using Microsoft Office Excel 2004

Note: The shaded numbers from '940' onwards are the set of twenty-five random numbers between '000' and '999' initially chosen; the numbers with an asterisk are the set of twenty-five random numbers between '000' and '499'.

different three-digit numbers between '000' and '999'. We are free *to choose any starting place* in the Table. Suppose we start at the 'cell' which is eleven rows down in the third column of cells: taking all three digits this gives us '940'. We are free to decide *to move in any direction*. Suppose we go down this column of cells, the next three digits are '891'. We continue in the same direction and get the sequence of three digit numbers '110', '416', '095'. Having reached the bottom of this column we can then choose to start at the top of the next column and so on, until we have the set of twenty-five numbers required (these are shown shaded). Each of these numbers identifies a nurse to be included in our simple random sample.

It is not always relevant to take *any* three digit number from the Table. For example, if our sampling frame holds a population of only five hundred nurses' names, then the number allocated to each name lies between '000' and '499'. Working from the same starting place in the Table, we see that the number '940', for example, does not now refer to any unit in the population; thus we cannot include *every possible* three-digit numbers from the table in our sample. In going down the chosen column of three digit numbers we take *only* those that lie between '000' and '499', omitting the rest. In this case we take the numbers shown with an asterisk in Table 3.1; we see that we actually go through more than fifty numbers to achieve the twenty-five we require.

When we identify each selected random number with the corresponding name, we obtain the set of twenty-five nurses which is our 'simple random sample'. There is no way to test such a sample to show that it is truly representative of the population because, by definition, we do not have the information about the population that we could test it against. We claim that it is a 'random sample' only by virtue of the process by which it is selected, and since it *is* a 'random sample' we know that it is just as likely to have been chosen as any other sample of the same size. But does this mean we may have picked an *unrepresentative* sample, just by chance? Unfortunately, this can be the case; for example our sample of twenty-five nurses may turn out to contain only female nurses under 25 years old. However, statistical methods try to mitigate such effects, by repeated sampling, etc. When a sample is randomly selected we are sure that at least it is not purposefully biased by the researcher for unscrupulous, improper reasons. More than this, we use the concept of random sampling to understand how a sample can be 'properly' selected; when this is the case the statistics from the sample allow us to provide estimates for the population parameters. This estimation is explored in more detail in Section 8.2.

Unfortunately, it is seldom easy to obtain a truly random sample of a human population and most research concerned with people is imperfect in this respect. The main problem is in forming an adequate sampling frame and in then ensuring that 100% response is obtained from the sample. Even studies of highly visible populations frequently depend on 'convenience samples'; for example, studies of patients very often recruit respondents sequentially when they are admitted to or discharged from hospital (as in

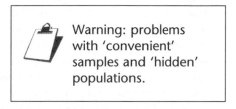

Warning: problems with 'convenient' samples and 'hidden' populations.

Coyle & Williams 2001). Then there are some human populations that are 'hidden', like drug users and prostitutes, and these pose particularly difficult sampling problems since sampling frames cannot be constructed (see Faugier & Sargeant 1997, Rhodes et al 1994, and Church et al 2001). When samples are not randomly selected then many statistical models cease to apply: the sample statistics are not in question and the conclusions may be true, but it is not always possible to extrapolate validly the findings from the sample and apply them to the population as a whole.

3.4 Other sampling procedures

The selection of simple random samples, especially when we require large samples from large populations, can turn out to be very time-consuming and costly. In practice there are many situations where we rely on modifications of the 'purely random' principle, and obtain samples by faster, cheaper, more organised methods. These samples are generally agreed to be sufficiently representative of the populations in question and, although they are not *perfectly* random, we do use them to provide statistics from which we estimate population parameters. The modifications are known as **sample designs**; among them are **stratified sampling, cluster sampling, multistage sampling** and **systematic sampling** – each of which we outline below.

Stratified sampling involves dividing the population of interest into sub sets known as 'strata' (that is, 'layers') and then sampling randomly within each layer or stratum. The number of units we take from each stratum should reflect the proportion of that stratum to the whole population. For example, to select a sample of hospital based nurses in a region we could begin by dividing the population by grade, that is into staff nurses, charge nurses, senior managers, etc., and we then take a simple random sample from each of these sub-sets. Of course, the acceptability of results obtained in this way depends upon the nature of the strata used.

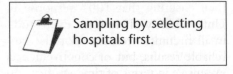

Sampling by nursing grade.

Cluster sampling involves the allocation of the units in a population into (equally sized) subsets called clusters. Then we apply a randomised procedure to select a sample of clusters. The overall 'cluster sample' then consists of all the units in the selected sample of clusters. An example of cluster sampling is first to take a random sample of the hospitals in the region (we assume the hospitals are of roughly the same size) and then to regard *every* nurse employed in those selected hospital as units in the cluster sample. Cluster sampling delivers a sample which might not be as representative of the population as we would like, but its major advantage is financial – by this method great savings can be made in the costs of data collection.

Sampling by selecting hospitals first.

The principle behind **multistage sampling** is that random selection occurs on at least two (possibly more) occasions. For example, in selecting a sample of nurses the first stage could be to select a random sample of hospitals in the region, and the second stage could then be to select a random sample of nurses from all those employed at each of the chosen hospitals. This sampling design is less likely than a simple random sample is to deliver a sample that is truly representative of the overall population – but it is fairly economical and it is commonly applied in national surveys.

Sampling by *selecting* nurses from a *selection* of hospitals.

Systematic sampling involves selecting units that are 'equally spaced' in the list of the population. If the population is listed in 'random order', then the result is a truly random sample. More usually the population has a 'natural' order, such as by age, alphabetical by surname, or by date of hospital admission: in these cases the ordering may well introduce some bias, and so we

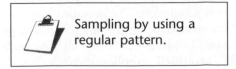

Sampling by using a regular pattern.

do not arrive at a truly random sample. As an example, suppose we wish to use this method to select a sample of twenty-five nurses from a population of one hundred nurses. We start by allocating a number between '1' and '100' to the name of each nurse. Dividing the size of the sample by the size of the population gives '25 ÷ 100', that is '¼', so we see that we shall be choosing 'one in four' of the population. To obtain a starting position in the population list, we toss a die or use Random Number Tables to get a number between '1' and '4': let us say we get '3'. Then we start with the 3rd number in the list, and subsequently choose every 4th number. The sequence we get is: 3rd, 7th, 11th, 15th, 19th, 23rd, and so on. The names which correspond to each of these numbers (from the 3rd to the 99th) give us the twenty-five nurses in our sample.

3.5 How big should a sample be?

Unfortunately, there is no easy answer to this question – one that is applicable in all circumstances. Intuitively it seems obvious that larger samples give more reliable results, but of course gathering large quantities of data is likely to be expensive in terms of time, money and convenience. Thus researchers are often limited in the sizes of the samples they use by considerations arising from the organisation and funding of their work.

None the less there are many features that should, if possible, be taken into account when deciding the size of a sample. The nature of the statistical problem is relevant (perhaps we want to estimate the population mean from our sample data? or perhaps we want to see if groups of people are significantly different from each other in some respect?), as is the population variability of the effect being studied, which we may already know from other studies or from preliminary work. Before we undertake a sampling procedure, in designing our statistical approach we should ideally decide on the 'level of confidence' and the 'level of significance' we wish our results to have, and the 'level of power' chosen for the study; these issues, discussed in Chapters 7, 8 and 9, may affect the sample size we choose. Accuracy in estimating the parameter of a population is determined just as much by careful design and execution of the research as by the size of sample: large samples by themselves do not guarantee the accuracy of results.

Presenting Data

4

– using tables and diagrams to summarise and display

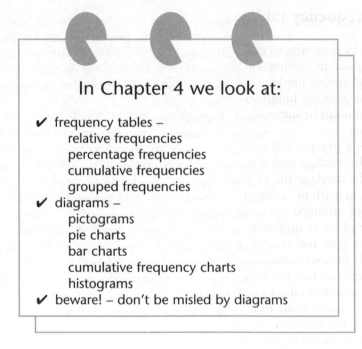

In Chapter 4 we look at:

✔ frequency tables –
   relative frequencies
   percentage frequencies
   cumulative frequencies
   grouped frequencies
✔ diagrams –
   pictograms
   pie charts
   bar charts
   cumulative frequency charts
   histograms
✔ beware! – don't be misled by diagrams

Tables and diagrams are increasingly part of daily life. We often see them illustrating issues in the media – for example graphing how prices have gone up in a certain timeframe, or showing the lengths of patient waiting lists in particular areas, or comparing the hours of sunshine in different holiday resorts. Tables and graphs are also very commonly used to illustrate results from clinical and healthcare research, and they are a tool in decision making for healthcare management.

So that we can understand the information to be obtained from tables, diagrams and graphs, we now look at how some of them are constructed. We assume that we have collected data (at appropriate levels of measurement) from relevant samples: when we have the lists of raw data our next job is to make sense of them! Here we shall deal with methods of **descriptive statistics**, and show how sets of numerical data can be turned into easily understood presentations using tables, diagrams and graphs.

The manipulations and presentations we use can easily be done on the many spreadsheet, database and statistical packages available for computers. But no matter how sophisticated the software, it should still be 'driven' by someone who understands the processes involved – to avoid nonsensical results. The last thing we want is the notorious 'GIGO' = 'Garbage In, Garbage Out'!

4.1 Frequency tables

We start by returning to the data set in Table 2.5 which is produced from the questionnaire in Section 2.3 and we find ourselves looking at an apparently incomprehensible jumble of numbers. In real-life quantitative research, a data set might be many hundreds of times bigger than this, but, even so, we now show that it can be summarised and presented in ways which can be understood at a glance.

As a first step towards organising a data set we arrange it into either **ascending or descending order**: this helps our understanding. We look at 'Nursing grade', the third variable in Table 2.5.
In the top part of Table 4.1 these figures are arranged (in columns) in the same order as originally given; in the lower part the same figures are arranged in ascending order. We

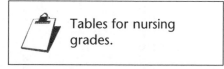

Tables for nursing grades.

immediately see that the lowest value is 4 (grade D), so it is obvious that there are no respondents from grades A, B or C. In addition, while the numerals 4, 5, 6 and 7 occur many times, there are fewer 8s and 9s; thus there are fewer respondents in the more senior grades H and I.

The information regarding 'Nursing grade' can be made more compact if we construct a **frequency table** for this variable, as shown in Table 4.2. A frequency table gives the total number of times each value or category occurs, that is, the **frequency** with which each occurs. Each coded value for a nursing grade is represented by the **symbol 'x'**, and the number of times each value occurs is represented by the **symbol 'f'** (for 'frequency'). When we read 'x', we ask ourselves '*what value* are we considering?'. When we read 'f', we ask ourselves '*how many times* does it occur?'. Since the value '4' occurs 34 times, the first row of the frequency table shows 'x = 4' and 'f = 34'; and so on. As a check, when we add up all the frequencies we get '120', which is the total

Table 4.1　Nursing grade, in original and ascending orders

					Original order						
6	6	6	5	7	5	7	7	8	7	4	5
4	7	5	9	5	4	8	4	4	4	6	4
7	6	4	8	5	4	5	7	7	6	6	4
6	9	7	5	5	4	4	6	5	6	5	6
5	7	8	7	6	4	7	4	6	7	6	4
5	5	9	6	9	4	5	8	7	4	6	5
4	5	8	4	5	6	7	4	6	7	4	6
4	6	7	4	8	4	5	5	4	4	6	5
4	4	5	4	8	4	9	4	8	5	6	5
5	7	7	4	4	6	8	5	7	6	6	4
					Ascending order						
4	4	4	4	5	5	6	6	6	7	7	8
4	4	4	4	5	5	6	6	6	7	7	8
4	4	4	4	5	5	6	6	6	7	7	8
4	4	4	4	5	5	6	6	6	7	7	8
4	4	4	5	5	5	6	6	6	7	7	8
4	4	4	5	5	5	6	6	7	7	8	9
4	4	4	5	5	5	6	6	7	7	8	9
4	4	4	5	5	5	6	6	7	7	8	9
4	4	4	5	5	5	6	6	7	7	8	9
4	4	4	5	5	5	6	6	7	7	8	9

Table 4.2　Nursing grade — frequency table

Grade	Value (x)	Number of values (f)
D	4	34
E	5	26
F	6	25
G	7	20
H	8	10
I	9	5
		total = n = 120

number of respondents. It is common to use the **symbol 'n'** to denote the total of all the frequencies: here 'n = 120'. A frequency table lets us see the whole data set at a glance.

It is often useful to extend frequency tables in different ways. If we wish, we can introduce a column for **relative frequency** and so construct a **relative frequency table** (see Table 4.3). A relative frequency expresses the frequency as a *fraction (or decimal) of the total frequency*, thus:

$$\text{relative frequency} = \frac{\textit{frequency}}{\textit{total frequency}}$$

Table 4.3   Nursing grade – relative frequency table

Grade	Value (x)	Frequency (f)	Relative frequency
D	4	34	$\dfrac{34}{120} = 0.28$
E	5	26	0.22
F	6	25	0.21
G	7	20	0.17
H	8	10	0.08
I	9	5	0.04
		n = 120	total = 1

(the relative frequencies are shown correct to 2 places of decimals)

We are still dealing with the nursing grades, so we know that the total frequency is 120, hence in this case:

$$\text{relative frequency} = \frac{frequency}{120}$$

As we see in Table 4.3, the total of all the relative frequencies relating to a sample is 'one'. We shall return to this idea of relative frequencies again in Chapter 7, when we consider probabilities.

Table 4.4   Nursing grade – percentage frequency table

Grade	Value (x)	Frequency (f)	Percentage frequency (%f)
D	4	34	$\dfrac{34}{120} \times 100\% = 28\%$
E	5	26	22%
F	6	25	21%
G	7	20	17%
H	8	10	8%
I	9	5	4%
		n = 120	total = 100%

(the percentage frequencies are shown correct to the nearest 1%)

We can also extend a frequency table by including a column for **percentage frequency (%f)**. For a **percentage frequency table** (as illustrated in Table 4.4) we write each frequency as *a percentage of the total frequency*. Thus:

$$\text{percentage frequency} = \frac{frequency}{total\ frequency} \times 100\%$$

In this case of Nursing Grades we know n = 120, and so

$$\text{percentage frequency} = \frac{frequency}{120} \times 100\%$$

We can also think of this as:

percentage frequency = relative frequency × 100%

and we see that the total of all the percentage frequencies relating to a sample is '100%'.

In addition, we can extend the frequency table to show **cumulative frequencies**. For this 'Nursing grade' example (see Table 4.5) the cumulative frequency column, or **cum-f** column, shows the total frequencies *up to and including* the value of x indicated. For 'x = 4' we see that the total number of occurrences up to and including 'x = 4' is '34'. For the next row in the table we count the number of occurrences up to and including the value 'x = 5'; it is '34 + 26' i.e. '60', so for 'x = 5' we have 'cum-f = 60'. For the next row we have 'x = 6' and the total of all the frequencies up to and including this value is '34 + 26 + 25 = 85'. For the cum-f entry, each time we add on the next frequency figure. As a check, the *final* entry in the cum-f column will *always* be the total of all the frequencies (n), that is – in this case – the total number of all the respondents.

Table 4.5   Nursing grade — cumulative frequency table

Value (x)	Frequency (f)	Cumulative frequency (cum-f)
4	34	34
5	26	60
6	25	85
7	20	105
8	10	115
9	5	120
	n = 120	

From a cumulative frequency table we can often detect patterns within the data. For example from Table 4.5 we immediately see that half of the respondents (60) are in Grades D and E, while more than 100 of the 120 are in Grade G or lower.

It is straightforward to extend Table 4.5 to show **percentage cumulative frequencies**. We calculate each figure shown in the cum-f column as a percentage of the total of all the frequencies, see Table 4.6. The total in this case is 'n = 120' and the calculations are straightforward.

When a variable takes *very many different values*, its frequency table might contain so many rows that it does not help our immediate understanding at all. This is the situation when we look at the results from Question 2 of the questionnaire (see Table 2.5). There are 33 different ages quoted, between 21 and 58 years old; the rather less-than-informative frequency table is shown in Table 4.7.

Table 4.6 Nursing grade – percentage frequency table

Value (x)	frequency (f)	Cum-f	Percentage cum-f
4	34	34	$\dfrac{34}{120} \times 100\% = 28\%$
5	26	60	50%
6	25	85	71%
7	20	105	88%
8	10	115	96%
9	5	120	100%
	n = 120		

(the percentage frequencies are shown correct to the nearest 1%)

Table 4.7 Nurses' ages – frequency table

Age (x)	Frequency (f)
21	2
22	4
23	1
24	3
25	4
26	5
27	9
28	6
29	2
30	7
31	6
32	7
33	6
34	5
35	4
36	3
37	6
38	3
39	5
41	3
42	5
43	1
44	2
46	4
47	2
48	2
49	2
51	2
52	2
53	3
55	1
56	2
58	1
	n = 120

Tables for grouping
nurses' ages; boundaries
on the birthdays.

To make more sense of these data we construct a **grouped frequency table**, grouping the values of the variable into convenient **bands** or **classes**. Instead of considering 'age' as a discrete variable, with separate ages recorded, 21 or 27 or 46, etc., we can consider it as a continuous variable, recorded in years and any fraction of a year (we are still measuring at ratio level). We might record the frequencies in five-year age bands, starting with 'How many nurses are 20 or over, but not yet 25?'; the answer is '10'. Then we ask 'How many nurses are 25 years or over, but not yet 30?'; the answer is '26'. And so on, until we ask 'How many nurses are 55 years or over, but not yet 60?'; the answer is '4'. We now tabulate this information in Table 4.8. Because everyone changes their stated age *actually on their birthday*, we notice that the **boundaries** between the bands are at 20 years old, 25 years old, 30 years old, etc. We write '20 or over, but not yet 25' as '20–(25)': the age of 'exactly 25' does not fall in this band, it just marks the boundary. If the upper boundary is obvious from the next band, then we can write '20–(25)' as '20–'. We *never* leave an 'open-ended' band; so we do not write '55 +' for the last of these bands, but rather '55–(60)' – *assuming* the final upper boundary where necessary.

Table 4.8   Nurses' ages – grouped frequency table (5 year band-widths)

Age band (x)	Frequency (f)
20–(25)	10
25–(30)	26
30–(35)	31
35–(40)	21
40–(45)	11
45–(50)	10
50–(55)	7
55–(60)	4
	n = 120

We choose the sizes of the classes, or bands, according to what is convenient or most useful. For example, we can group the nurses' ages into ten-year bands as shown in Table 4.9, or even into bands of unequal width as shown in Table 4.10. When we group data like this we notice that when we have *many* bands we may have a cluttered diagram, but when we have *too few* bands we may actually be losing a lot of the detail.

As discussed above, when we are dealing with ages the **class boundaries** clearly occur *at the birthdays*. However, in practice, there are many situations where class boundaries do not occur on 'whole numbers'. Suppose, for example,

Table 4.9 Nurses' ages – grouped frequency table
(10 year band-widths)

Age band (x)	Frequency (f)
20–(30)	36
30–(40)	52
40–(50)	21
50–(60)	11
	n = 120

Table 4.10 Nurses' ages – grouped frequency table
(unequal band-widths)

Age band (x)	Frequency (f)
20–(30)	36
30–(35)	31
35–(40)	21
40–(60)	32
	n = 120

we are measuring the weight loss of different people under a certain dietary regime: our data set is a list of weights, expressed in kilograms to the nearest 0.1 of a kilogram. We can group these weights into classes, roughly zero to 1 kg, 1 kg to 2 kg,

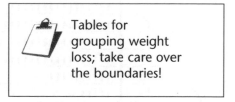

Tables for grouping weight loss; take care over the boundaries!

2 kg to 3 kg etc., but we must be very careful where the boundaries are. If we want the first class to contain all the weights *up to but not including* 1 kg, then its **upper boundary** is at '0.95 kg'. This is because the weights are recorded to the nearest 0.1 kg, so any weight between 0.95 kg and1 kg will 'round up' to 1kg. We now see that the **lower boundary** of the second class is '0.95 kg'; its upper boundary is at 1.95 kg, since any weight between 0.95 kg and 2 kg is recorded as '2 kg'; and so on for each class. When grouping the frequencies of a continuous variable, where each piece of data is inevitably subject to some 'rounding', we must consider carefully the position of each class boundary.

4.2 Diagrams for data

Tables like the ones above are an excellent way to order and present data, but for immediate impact we turn to **graphical representations**. Here we look at just five ways to present data using diagrams: we look at **pictograms**, **pie charts**, **bar charts**, **cumulative frequency charts** and **histograms** (in increasing order of sophistication). Pictograms, pie charts and bar charts are used for displaying data from *discrete variables*; histograms can *only* be used with *continuous variables*. Cumulative frequency charts can be drawn for either type of data: when using discrete data we get a **cumulative bar chart**, or a **cumulative frequency (cum-f) polygon** made up of straight lines; when using continuous data we more commonly get a **cumulative frequency (cum-f) curve** known as an **ogive**.

The simplest forms of diagrams are called **pictograms**. In these we use a particular symbol, called an **ideogram**, to represent a particular occurrence of the value or category. This type of presentation is often used in the mass media – it is easy to do, with clipart-type symbols readily available from the internet. However, the artwork can distract from the message being conveyed, it can be unappealing or introduce inaccuracies. There are some other drawbacks to pictograms, as we shall see. Using an ideogram to represent each nurse, we can illustrate the data on 'Nursing grade' (see Table 4.2) by the pictogram in Figure 4.1.

Nursing grades: pictograms.

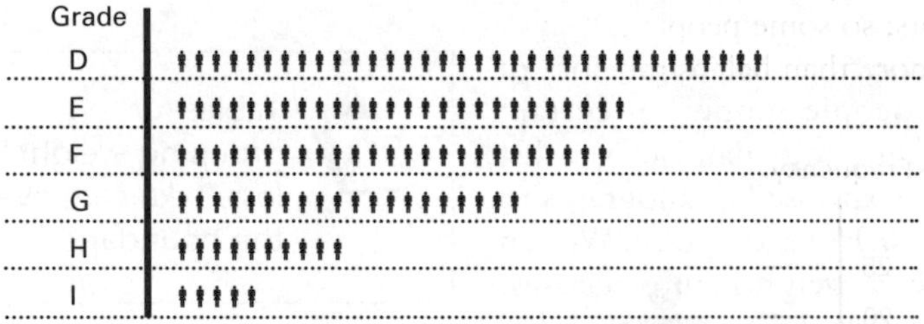

Figure 4.1   Pictogram to show nursing grades (n = 120)

Pictograms are used to display frequencies of values where the variable has been measured at a nominal or an ordinal level, but they can be cumbersome, with very long rows of symbols. In fact, with one symbol for each item, Figure 4.1 is a version of a **tally chart** (where a tick or a stroke 'counts' each occurrence). To show the information more efficiently we could use one ideogram to represent a larger frequency, of say '3' (including this fact in the key). This makes the rows shorter and easier to read and compare, see Figure 4.2. However, the extra '1s' and '2s', where, for instance:

$$'34 = (11 \times 3) + 1'$$
$$\text{and } '26 = (8 \times 3) + ②'$$

are hard to illustrate!

A third way to present a pictogram is by allowing the *height* of each ideogram to represent the frequency. Thus a shape *half* as tall as another would represent

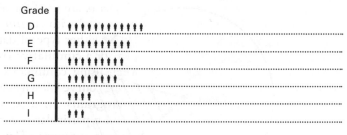

Key: ✝ = 3 nurses

Figure 4.2   Another pictogram showing nursing grades (n = 120)

a frequency just *half* of the other, and so on. The information on Grades F and G (frequencies '25' and '20' respectively) could be shown as in Figure 4.3. A drawback here is that our eyes naturally compare areas rather

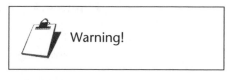

Warning!

than heights; so some people might, incorrectly, take this diagram to show that there are more than half as many nurses again in Grade F as in Grade G.

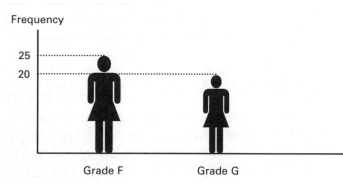

Figure 4.3   A pictogram comparing numbers in grades F and G

A **pie chart** represents frequencies in a circle, which we imagine to be sliced up like a pie or a pizza. Each 'slice' of a pie touches the centre of the circle; this shape is called a **sector** of the circle (see Figure 4.4).

In a pie chart the frequencies of different values or categories are represented by the *areas of the corresponding sectors;* this makes a virtue of our greater ability to appreciate areas! It is a useful fact that the *area* of each sector is proportional to the *angle* it makes at the centre of the circle, so to construct a pie chart we need just to calculate the relevant angle corresponding to each frequency. Since there are 360° in a circle we use this method:

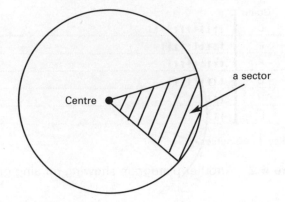

Figure 4.4   A sector of a circle

$$\text{angle at the centre} = \frac{frequency}{total\ frequency} \times 360°$$

Nursing grades:
pie charts.

For our 'Nursing grade' frequencies (Table 4.2), we show in Table 4.11 the angles in the sectors for each category. Figure 4.5 shows the resulting pie chart.

There are many computer packages that construct pie charts for us. If we need to draw one by hand it is a matter of using a pair of compasses (for the circle and its centre) and a protractor (for the angles).

Pie charts can always be used to represent frequencies of values or categories when a variable is measured at nominal or ordinal level, but they are most valuable when we wish to represent *constituent parts of a whole*, and see a *whole* picture of the proportions of the frequencies. From a pie chart we can immediately see

Table 4.11   Nursing grades, calculating the angles for the pie chart

Grade	Frequency (f)	Angle
D	34	$\frac{34}{120} \times 360° = 102°$
E	26	78°
F	25	75°
G	20	60°
H	10	30°
I	5	15°
	n = 120	total = 360°

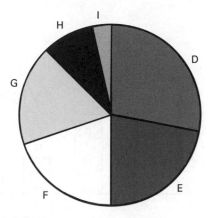

Figure 4.5 Pie chart showing nursing grades

just how big the sectors are relative to each other. From Figure 4.5 we see easily that the Grade D nurses form almost one third of the respondents, and that just less than one quarter of the nurses are in Grade F.

Computer packages often offer us various elaborations upon a basic pie chart. These can include expanding selected sectors for special note, or drawing a three-dimensional version of the chart. Perhaps these appear attractive from an artistic point of view, but it is normally *not* good practice to use them. The reason is that they *distort* the apparent proportions of the sectors. In Figure 4.6 we illustrate this: since our eyes 'take in' volumes

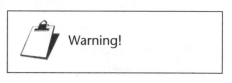

even better than they see areas, at first sight it seems that there are about twice as many Grade E nurses than Grade G nurses – but we know that this is false!

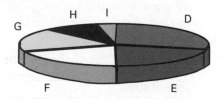

Figure 4.6 3-D pie chart showing nursing grades

A **(simple) bar chart** is a way of displaying data where the **length of a bar** (or column) represents the frequency of the value or category. Usually the bars are drawn vertically and the **height** of each is measured with reference to a fixed vertical line marked with a scale, as a ruler is. This vertical line is called the **y-axis**, and the zero point on it is called the **origin**. The bars are arranged parallel with the

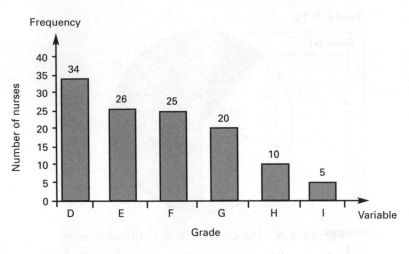

Figure 4.7   Bar chart showing nursing grades

y-axis, 'standing' on a horizontal line called the **x-axis** which passes through the origin. All the individual bars have the same width, and (ideally) they are always separated from each other by a similar width of gap. Along the x-axis we label the value or category represented by each bar; the variable can be measured at nominal, ordinal or interval level. The heights of the bars, and hence the frequencies they indicate, can easily be compared. Using the data from Table 4.2, Figure 4.7 shows a bar chart indicating the numbers of nurses, i.e. the frequencies, in each of the grades.

Nursing grades:
bar chart.

Presented like this, the data have an immediate impact. From Figure 4.7 it is obvious that nurses in the D grade form the largest group, and those in the I grade form the smallest. We easily see the overall situation that there are relatively fewer nurses in the more senior grades.

As another example of a bar chart we look at the variable 'nurse satisfaction', dealt with in Question 6 of the questionnaire (Table 2.2). From Table 2.5, we first lift the figures from the column labelled 'satis' and construct the frequency table shown, Table 4.12. Even though the values in Table 4.12 are numerical, they are distinct (we have a discrete variable) so we draw a bar chart as in Figure 4.8 to illustrate their frequencies.

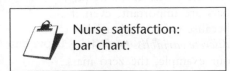

Nurse satisfaction:
bar chart.

We can note some important features of bar charts. The axes show the level of measurement applicable to the variable being plotted. In the case of Figure 4.7

Table 4.12   Nurse satisfaction – a frequency table

Score (x)	Frequency (f)
1	4
2	9
3	13
4	18
5	23
6	24
7	13
8	7
9	6
10	3
	n = 120

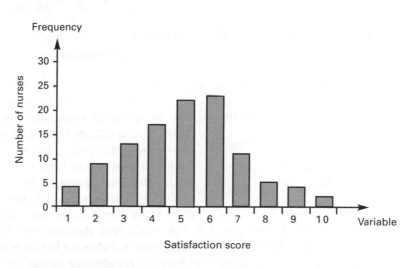

Figure 4.8   Bar chart showing nurse satisfaction

the horizontal x-axis shows 'Nursing grade' measured at ordinal level, and the vertical y-axis shows the frequency ('How many nurses?') measured at ratio level. In Figure 4.8 the x-axis shows 'Nurse satisfaction' measured at interval level, and the y-axis shows frequency measured at ratio level. The gaps between the bars are important, even if the values of the variable are numerical: this is because we can *only* use bar charts for *discrete variables*. As we have shown in our example, the zero mark (origin) on the y-axis should *always* be shown and we should draw every bar to its *full scale height*; failure to do these things can lead to very misleading results (see Section 4.3).

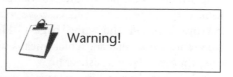

Warning!

As well as simple bar charts, which show the frequency of each value separately,

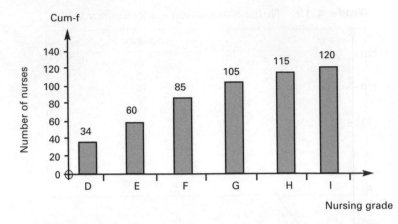

Figure 4.9   Cumulative bar chart showing nurses' grades

we can draw **cumulative bar charts**. This presentation can only be used for a variable which is measured at an ordinal level (or higher). Just as with a (simple) bar chart, the values of the variable are indicated in order along the x-axis, the scale on the y-axis indicates the frequency of each and equally spaced bars of equal width are used. From the figures in Table 4.5, we can draw the cumulative bar chart shown in Figure 4.9. We can 'say' the information from this diagram in different ways: as '*up to and including* Grade F there are 85 nurses', or, 'the frequency of nurses *up to and including* grade F is 85' or 'the *total number* of nurses *up to and including* Grade F is 85'.

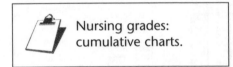

Nursing grades: cumulative charts.

We can simplify the presentation of a cumulative bar chart by joining the mid-points of the tops of the bars by straight lines (see Figure 4.10). If we then dispense with the actual bars we have a **cumulative frequency polygon**. We note that a cum-f polygon should always be drawn to begin on the x-axis, by inventing a 'previous' value with zero frequency if necessary.

In contrast with all the types of diagrams used so far, a **histogram** displays data concerning a *continuous variable*. If we draw a standard bar chart for a variable which takes many different values (see Table 4.7), then the diagram can look very cluttered (in this case we would need to construct thirty-three very narrow bars on the same page!). However, if we work from a grouped frequency table instead, which means we are taking the variable to be continuous, then we draw a histogram.

Like a bar chart, a histogram is drawn using a (vertical) y-axis and a (horizontal) x-axis, which meet at the origin. As before the y-axis is marked with a scale, like on a ruler, and on a histogram the x-axis is *also* marked with a ruler-like

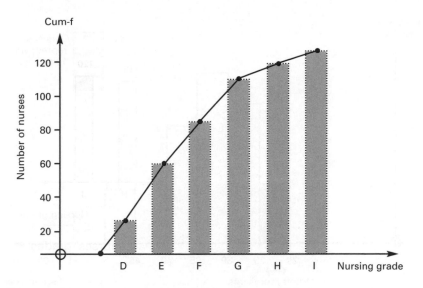

Figure 4.10   Cumulative frequency polygon showing nurses' grades

scale: the origin is the *joint zero point* on both *axes*. Thus on both axes we can indicate measurements at an interval or a ratio level; on the scales we can indicate *any* whole number or *any* fraction or decimal in-between whole numbers.

We now use the figures from Table 4.8 to draw a histogram for the variable 'Nurses' ages', remembering that this is *only* possible because 'age' is here considered to be a continuous variable. The result is shown in Figure 4.11. We see that indicating the grouped frequency for each age band, or class, gives us a rectangle on the diagram and these rectangles are of equal width because the age bands are equal. As on *all* histograms, the *rectangles actually touch* each other; this is essential because the x-axis represents a continuous variable, so *no gaps* are possible.

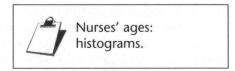

Nurses' ages: histograms.

Another important feature of a histogram is that the frequencies are actually represented by the *areas of the rectangles* (rather that by their heights). We remember the basic formula:

area of a rectangle = its height × its width

When the band-widths are equal (in this case they are all five years), we consider each band-width to be 'one unit' and then we use the given scale on the y-axis (see Figure 4.11) to calculate the areas. On a histogram the y-axis actually measures **frequency density**. Each histogram is accompanied by a **key**, which shows how the areas are related to the frequencies.

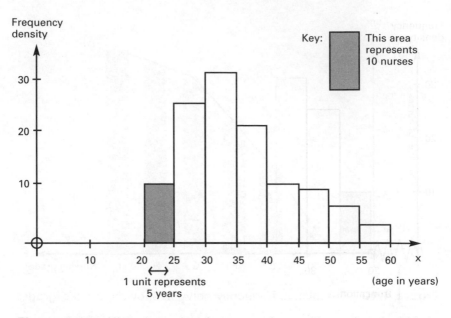

Figure 4.11 Histogram showing nurses' ages (5 year band-widths)

We may wish to show this histogram more clearly by 'truncating' the x-axis so that the important part of the diagram is more prominent: we must always indicate this clearly, as shown in Figure 4.12.

Using the figures from Table 4.9, we can draw a different histogram for 'Nurses' ages'. In Figure 4.13 we show this; each 'unit' along the x-axis here indicates the band-width of ten years, so when we use the given scale on the y-axis the areas of the rectangles represent the frequencies.

We can draw yet another histogram for 'Nurses' ages' by using the figures from Table 4.10: here the band-widths are *not* all equal. In Figure 4.14 we indicate how we must choose a particular band-width to be 'one unit' – we choose 'five years' in this case – and then we use the scale on the y-axis (more carefully!) to make the area of each rectangle represent the frequency.

Sometimes, to 'guide the eye', it is useful to join the mid-points of the tops of the rectangles in a histogram with straight lines. Figure 4.15 shows this adaption of Figure 4.13. The result is a **frequency polygon** and we note that the polygon is always completed by drawing lines which join it to the x-axis (by imagining extra classes with zero frequency to left and right). The area *beneath the polygon* indicates the total frequency (this is *exact* when the classes are equal, but approximate when the classes are unequal).

We can also draw the **cumulative frequency polygon** which corresponds to any histogram. An important feature of this is that each 'cum-f' point must be plotted at the *upper boundary* of the class concerned, since it

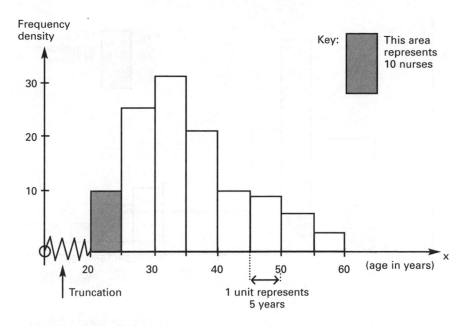

Figure 4.12   Histogram showing nurses' ages (5 year band-widths)
showing the truncation

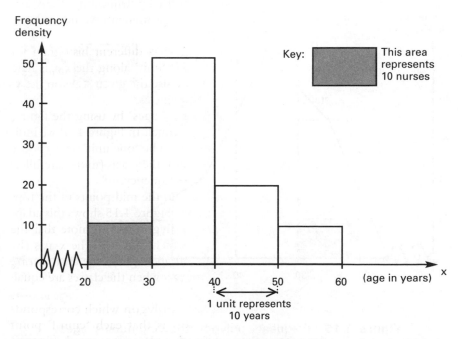

Figure 4.13   Histogram showing nurses' ages (10 year band-widths)

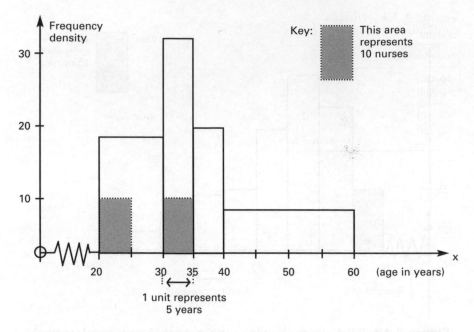

Figure 4.14   Histogram showing nurses' ages (unequal band-widths)

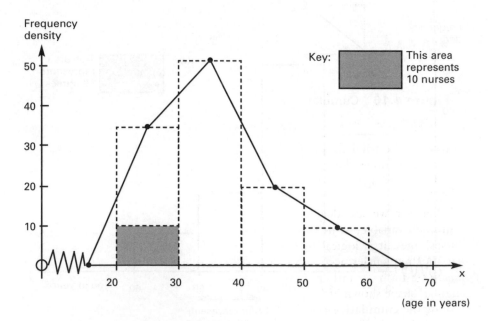

Figure 4.15   Frequency polygon showing nurses' ages
(10 year band-widths)

Table 4.13 Nurses' ages – grouped frequency table for graphing cumulative frequencies (10 year band-widths)

Age band (x)	Frequency (f)	Cum-f	Upper bound
10–(20)	0	0	20
20–(30)	36	36	30
30–(40)	52	88	40
40–(50)	21	109	50
50–(60)	11	120	60
	n = 120		

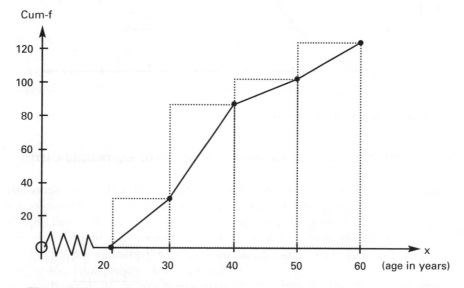

Figure 4.16 Cumulative frequency polygon showing nurses' ages

represents the total frequency *up to and including the whole* of that class. Figure 4.16 shows the cumulative frequency polygon based on Table 4.13, for the Nurses' ages in 10 year band-widths.

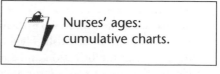

Nurses' ages: cumulative charts.

Whenever we are dealing with a *continuous* variable, as in this case of Nurses' ages, it is logical to suppose that the frequencies accumulate in a *smooth* fashion – rather than the 'angular' shape shown in Figure 4.16. Thus from Table 4.13 we are more likely to draw the **cumulative frequency curve** shown in Figure 4.17. This is called an **ogee**-shaped curve, or an **ogive**.

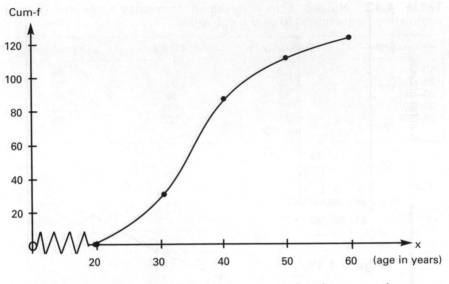

Figure 4.17 Cumulative frequency curve showing nurses' ages

4.3 Graphical presentations: informing or misleading?

Many charts, diagrams and graphs which display statistical data are rigorously constructed and convey information easily and straightforwardly. However it *is* possible to misuse statistical approaches to give a deliberately distorted impression of the facts. We have already mentioned, in Section 4.2, that several types of pictograms and three-dimensional pie-charts in particular are capable of giving false impressions. Now we consider a variety of ploys which can be applied to bar charts and histograms for the purpose of modifying the impression given. These can be quite simple amendments: they do not necessarily amount to presenting false information, but rather they tend to take the unwary 'for a walk up the garden path'.

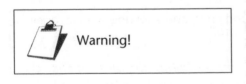

Warning!

The bar chart in Figure 4.18 shows the annual number of new HIV infections reported in a Scottish Health Board area between 1981 and 1994 (Scottish Centre for Infection and Environmental Health (SCIEH) 1995). We see clearly that there was a large increase in the number of new infections in 1984, attributable to needle sharing among injecting drug users. In the following years the numbers of new infections declined as a result of public health interventions such as needle exchanges and health education. Even a cursory glance at the diagram sees that the epidemic was coming under control towards the end of the 1980s.

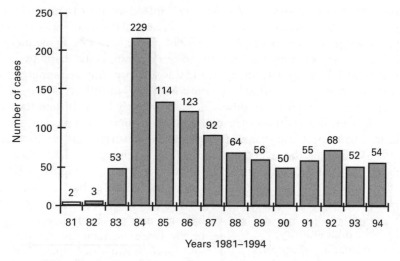

Figure 4.18 Bar chart showing new HIV infections

Suppose that we have a hidden agenda: we wish to show that the public health measures had little effect and that the epidemic continued to rage. We can change the impression given by the data by altering the presentation. Figure 4.19 illustrates exactly the same data as shown in Figure 4.18, only this time we present it as a cumulative frequency bar chart.

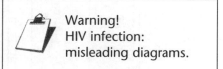

Warning!
HIV infection:
misleading diagrams.

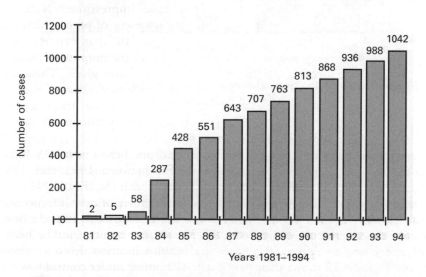

Figure 4.19 Cumulative frequency bar chart: HIV infections

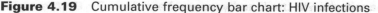

Because the bars in Figure 4.19 show '*total* infections up to and including 1988' etc., we see how there is a fairly steep rise in each of the first four years, with the rise continuing, but not so steeply, until 1994. As we have already mentioned, our eyes 'take in' areas better than heights, so this diagram could easily sway the unsuspecting into thinking that the epidemic was still spreading alarmingly.

Bar charts can also be modified by combining bars in different ways or by truncating the y-axis. If these modifications are properly labelled then they are legitimate devices, but even so they can be used to mislead someone who is not prepared to inspect the diagram carefully. To illustrate this we look at a hypothetical example: the average numbers of bed sheets used weekly by medical and surgical specialties in a NHS Trust hospital. In Figure 4.20 we

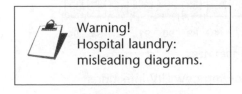

show the simple bar chart. The general medical unit is clearly the heaviest user of clean sheets; it uses nearly twice as many as the surgical unit, and almost three times as many as the ENT unit.

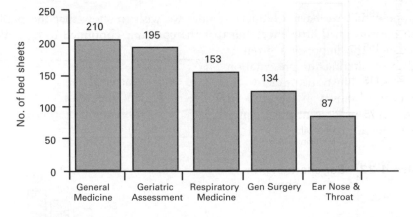

Figure 4.20   Bar chart: average bed sheet use by medical and surgical specialties

We suppose that laundry resources are going to be cut back on the basis of this information. Since the person who draws the chart is the one who decides its layout, the surgical and ENT units may decide to combine their returns and produce a new chart, as in Figure 4.21.

This shows a very different picture: the general surgery and ENT units are the heaviest users of linen and the medical unit has been put into second place. We would now suppose that, faced with this presentation, the medical unit will redraw the chart, to redress the score and ensure it continues to receive resources. Figure 4.22 shows their new chart. They truncate the scale on the y-axis (the scale starts at y = 75, the x-axis no longer goes through the origin) and

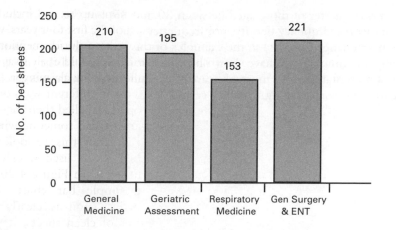

Figure 4.21 Bar chart: average bed sheet use by combined specialties

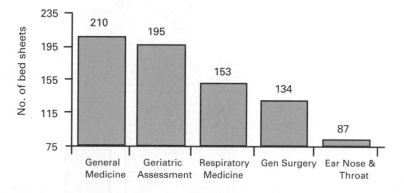

Figure 4.22 Bar chart: average bed sheet use by medical and surgical specialties (truncated axis)

now the use by general surgery and ENT looks tiny in comparison with that of the medical unit. This is a common way used to try to distort the impression given by a chart.

There are several ways that an accurate presentation in a histogram can be 'adjusted' to give a false impression. Among these are deceiving the eye by truncating the y-axis, which works just as described above for a bar chart. Inaccuracies can also be implied by using the fact that on a histogram it is the *area* of each rectangle that represents the frequency involved. To illustrate this we look again at Figure 4.14: at a quick glance it might seem that the number of nurses between 55 and 60

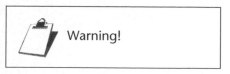

Warning!

is about one quarter of those aged between 30 and 35, but this is not so – the y-axis measures frequency density, not frequency.

We have changed no data in the examples of this section. However, without falsifying any numbers we have shown how easy it is to mislead the unwary by different presentations. We must take care to examine all presentations carefully, to identify the *real* meaning that they carry.

Summarising Data

5

– using numbers to represent key features of data sets

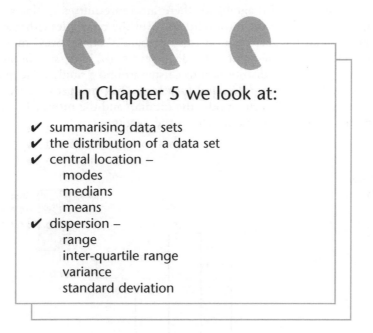

In Chapter 5 we look at:

✔ summarising data sets
✔ the distribution of a data set
✔ central location –
  modes
  medians
  means
✔ dispersion –
  range
  inter-quartile range
  variance
  standard deviation

It can be very challenging to be faced with a large quantity of data from a survey or a research project. We can start by organising it using frequency tables and then presenting it with different charts and diagrams. However, no matter how carefully these tables and graphs are prepared, they are sometimes not sufficiently informative. This is especially so if we are dealing with many variables, and so have an unwieldy number of charts to be compared.

The **distribution** of a data set means the overall relationship between the values of the variable and their frequencies; it is often called a **frequency**

distribution. A single chart can give a clear impression about the distribution of a single data set, but we often need to be able to compare distributions of different variables, maybe taken from different groups of respondents. It is not easy to make valid comparisons between different charts or graphs; so to compare distributions we use **summary (descriptive) statistics**.

5.1 The key summary statistics

Nurses' ages: an overview.

To give us insight into what summary statistics are, we return to the histogram of 'Nurses' ages' (Figure 4.11), redrawn here as Figure 5.1.

There is an obvious peak on this graph with the '30–(35)' age-band: there are more nurses in this age-group than any other, they are the most frequent. But the rectangles either side seem to cluster around the rectangle on this age-band, 'falling away' more or less regularly. Thus the age-band '30–(35)' seems to have significance. This tendency of a frequency distribution to cluster around a single value or band of values is called a tendency to **central location**. The principal ways we measure central location are called the **mode**, the **median** and the **mean** (this last is the 'arithmetic' mean, known informally as the **average**).

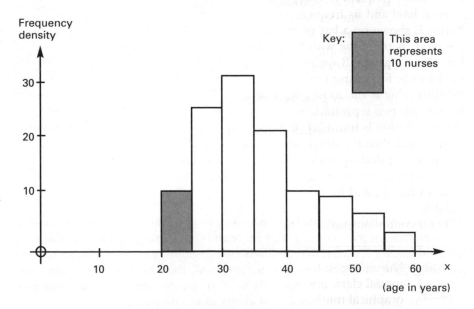

Figure 5.1   Histogram of nurses' ages (as Figure 4.11)
(5 year band-widths)

In addition, in Figure 5.1 we see that the values of the variable are 'spread out' along the (horizontal) x-axis, between the ages '20' and '60' but with more values at the younger end. Exactly *how much* the values are spread out – what the limits are, whether the spread is even, if there are noticeable clusters, whether either end tails off to zero – identifies the **dispersion** of the distribution. The main measures of dispersion are the **range**, the **inter-quartile range**, the **variance** and the **standard deviation**.

Each measure of central location gives us a *single number* (or category) which we think of as representing the whole distribution; each measure of dispersion gives us a *single number* which describes the 'spread-out-ness' of the distribution. By comparing these numbers for different distributions we can compare the distributions themselves.

As we shall see, these measures of 'central location' and 'dispersion' come naturally grouped. The mode and the range are the simplest measures. The median and the inter-quartile range are used on variables at ordinal level or above. Means, variances and standard deviations are the most sophisticated measures, used on variables at interval or ratio level.

5.2 Central location: mode, median and mean

We start with the simplest measure of central location. The **mode** or **modal value** is the value (or category) of the variable which occurs most, that is, has the greatest frequency. When a variable is measured at nominal, ordinal or interval level and its frequency distribution is shown on a bar graph, then the mode is the value with the *tallest* bar. From Figure 4.8 we see that the modal value for 'Nurse satisfaction' is '6' (this value is the most common).

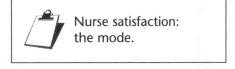

Nurse satisfaction: the mode.

If there are two separate bars which have equal maximum height, we say that the distribution is **bimodal**. If there are more than two bars with equal maximum height then the distribution is **multi-modal** (see Figure 5.2(a) and (b)). When we are dealing with discrete data, it is always easy to 'spot' the mode from a frequency table or a bar chart; it does not require us to do any calculations to find it, and its value is always one of the *actual values* taken by the variable.

For a continuous variable, measured at interval or ratio level, the frequency distribution is shown by a histogram. In this case we cannot read off the (single) modal value, but we can read off the **modal class** of the variable. Looking at Figure 5.1, we see that the modal class for the nurses' ages is the class '30–(35)'. In a case like this

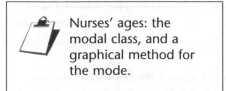

Nurses' ages: the modal class, and a graphical method for the mode.

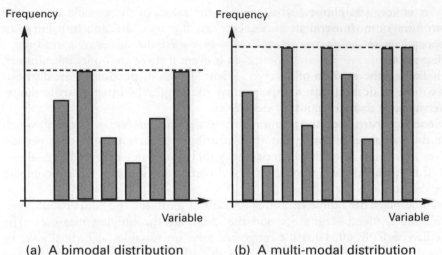

(a) A bimodal distribution   (b) A multi-modal distribution

Figure 5.2   Bar charts showing bimodal and multi-modal distributions

we can use a simple construction to get an estimate of the mode itself as a single number. We join the 'opposite corners' on the modal rectangle, as shown in Figure 5.3. The point where the lines cross indicates a value for the mode, so here the modal age is approximately '32'.

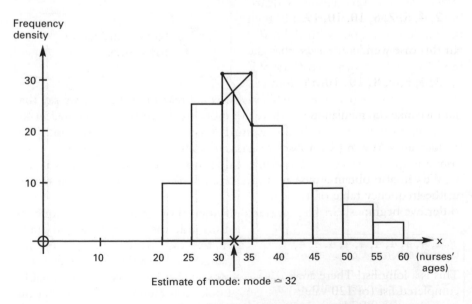

Figure 5.3   A graphical method to estimate a mode (based on the histogram of Figure 5.1)

It is very straightforward to obtain the mode, but is not considered the strongest or most useful measure of central tendency. This is because it does *not* depend on *the whole* data set, nor is it associated with any specific measure of dispersion.

To find the **median** of a data set, sometimes written with the **symbol 'M'**, we must be dealing with a variable which is measured at or above ordinal level. We imagine that all the instances of all the values of the variable are arranged *in ascending order*, then the median of the distribution is the value *in the middle*.

As a simple example, if we want the median of the values:

2, 10, 34, 5, 7, 17, 4, 8, 10

we first place the numbers in ascending order:

2, 4, 5, 7, 8, 10, 10, 19, 34

We have nine numbers here (n = 9) and 'nine' is an odd number, so the middle one is the fifth:

2, 4, 5, 7, ⑧, 10, 10, 19, 34

and thus the median of this set is 'M = 8'.

Of course sometimes we might have an even number of values. For the following set n = 10:

2, 4, 5, 7, 8, 10, 10, 19, 34, 35

In this case we identify *both* of the 'middle values' (here the fifth and sixth):

2, 4, 5, 7, ⑧, ⑩, 10, 19, 34, 35

and we take the median as mid-way (that is half-way) between these two. Thus:

median = M = ½ (8 + 10) = ½ × 18 = 9

We can also obtain a median value from a frequency table. If we look again at the frequency table of Table 4.2 and start to list all the values in ascending order, we begin:

4, 4, 4, 4, 4, 4, 4, 4, 4, 4, 4, 4, 4, 4, 4, etc.

This is a long list! There are 34 '4s', followed by 26 '5s', and so on. From the completed list (of 120 values) we must take the middle value (or the mid-way point between the two middle values). In fact it is easier to do this from the *cumulative frequency table*, Table 4.5, rewritten here as Table 5.1.

Table 5.1   Cumulative frequency table for nursing grades

Value (x)	Frequency (f)	Cumulative frequency (cum-f)
4	34	34
5	26	60
6	25	85
7	20	105
8	10	115
9	5	120
	n = 120	

There are a hundred and twenty values in the list altogether (n = 120). Because this is an even number the median is half way between the sixtieth and the sixty-first values. By inspecting the cum-f column, we see that the sixtieth value is '5' and the sixty-first value is '6', so for the nursing grades:

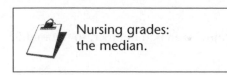

Nursing grades: the median.

$$\text{median} = M = \tfrac{1}{2}(5 + 6) = 5\tfrac{1}{2}$$

If we wish, we can generalise the reasoning used here. When there is an *odd number* of values in the data set – '*n*' *is odd* – the median is the ½(n + 1)th value. When there is an *even number* of values in the data set – '*n*' *is even* – then the median is half-way between the ½nth and the (½n + 1)th values.

When we are dealing with grouped data, and the size of the data set might be very large, often the simplest way to obtain an estimate for a median is from the cumulative frequency chart. Using the cum-f curve (for a continuous variable) we draw a horizontal line from the position on the y-axis which marks the 'middle-of-total-frequency'.

Nurses' ages: a graphical method for the median.

Where this cuts the curve shows us the median value for the variable. We illustrate this in Figure 5.4, from which we see that the median of the nurses' ages is approximately '36'.

The median is generally more useful than the mode. It is very easily calculated, but it does not depend on *every* value in the data set since values at the extremes of the distribution are ignored completely. We also notice that sometimes the median is not an actual value of the variable: this may or may not be a draw-back in different circumstances. The median is closely allied to two measures of dispersion: the range and the inter-quartile range.

Finally we come to the **mean** of a data set (more properly called the **arithmetic mean** – there are others) which in daily life is sometimes called the **average**. Means can only be determined when the variable is measured at interval or ratio level. In the simplest terms, the mean is calculated by *adding up all the*

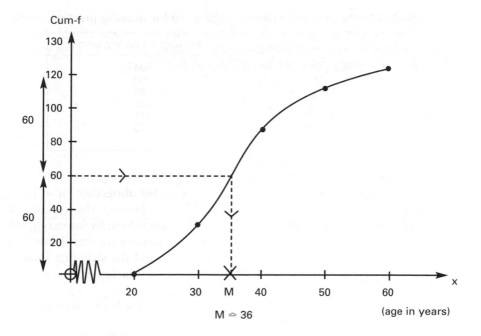

Figure 5.4 A graphical method to estimate a median
(based on the cum-f curve of Figure 4.17)

numbers in a data set then *dividing by how many of them there are*. As a simple example, to find the mean of the data set:

2, 10, 34, 5, 7, 19, 4, 8, 10

we add all these numbers together (the '10' occurs twice so it is included twice):

2 + 10 + 34 + 5 + 7 + 19 + 4 + 8 + 10 = 99

so the total is '99'. It is easy to count how many numbers there are, obviously 'nine' of them (n = 9). Thus for this data set:

$$\text{mean} = \frac{99}{9} = 11$$

To show more concisely how a mean is calculated, we can use some special symbols. Each value that a variable takes is represented by the letter 'x' (as in Section 4.1), and when we are dealing with a *sample* (see Section 3.2) the mean of the data set is denoted by the **symbol 'x̄'**, which we say as 'x bar'. In Statistics the **symbol 'Σ'** (which is pronounced '**sigma**' and is actually just the capital letter 'S' in the Greek alphabet) is used to indicate 'add them all up'. So the meaning of 'Σx' is 'add up all the values of "x"'. Remembering that the symbol 'n' denotes how many values we are dealing with, we have:

$$(\text{sample}) \text{ mean} = \bar{x} = \frac{\Sigma x}{n}$$

Using the numbers from Table 4.7 we can calculate the mean of all the Nurses' ages. Adding up all the separate ages $(21 + 21 + 22 + 22 + 22 + 22 + 23 + 24 + 24 + 24 + \text{etc.})$ gives:

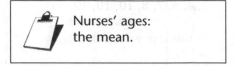
Nurses' ages:
the mean.

$$\Sigma x = 4173$$

so the mean age is

$$\bar{x} = \frac{\Sigma x}{n} = \frac{4173}{120} = 34.775$$

which is just over 34 years and 9 months.

The mean is the *strongest* of the measures of central tendency that we consider. *Every* value in the data set is involved when we calculate it, so the mean is particularly useful in detecting small differences between sets of data. Obviously, as in our examples above, the mean need not itself take a value of the variable; means are often calculated correct to several places of decimals. It is closely connected to the measures of dispersion known as *variance* and *standard deviation*.

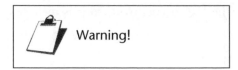
Warning!

There can sometimes be a drawback with the mean. If the data set consists only of a group of very high values together with a group of very low values, then the mean is a value nowhere near either group – this can give a distorted view of the whole distribution. To illustrate this we consider a group of patients of whom approximately half are aged about 80 and the rest are aged about 20. Calculation yields a mean value of around 50, but this age does *not* realistically represent the whole group!

5.3 Dispersion: ranges, variance and standard deviation

The simplest measure of dispersion is the overall **range**. This can be applied to variables at or above ordinal level. At its simplest (when the variable is measured at ordinal level) the range specifies '*from the least to the greatest*'. When the variable is measured at interval or ratio levels, the range is calculated as the *difference* between the largest value of the variable and the smallest. For the data set:

2, 10, 34, 5, 7, 17, 4, 8, 10

we place the numbers in ascending order, giving:

2, 4, 5, 7, 8, 10, 10, 19, 34

In this case we see that the range is 'from "2" to "34"', which we calculate as:

range = 34 − 2 = 32

We can obtain the range from a frequency table. From Table 4.7, the youngest nurse's age is '21' and the age of the oldest nurse is '58', so we have:

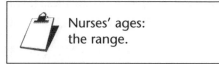
Nurses' ages: the range.

range = 58 − 21 = 37

Alternatively, the range can easily be read from the x-axis of a bar chart or a histogram: from the grouped data shown in Figure 5.1 the lowest age is '20' and the highest age is '60', so here:

range = 60 − 20 = 40

(The 'grouping' has caused us to lose some accuracy.)

The range gives us a 'ball-park' figure for the distribution. However, there are several reasons why it is not a completely satisfactory measure of dispersion: it is calculated on just two values of the data set, and ignores other features like 'bunching up' or 'extreme outliers'. For example, if we record the incomes of a group of student nurses over the last year, we might expect them all to be near to the level of a bursary plus the income from some part-time work. Suppose that one person in our group has won £100,000 from the Lottery: this makes the value of the range about £90,000, which is altogether misleading as a group descriptor!

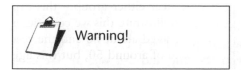
Warning!

To overcome the problem introduced by the inclusion of extreme values, we often calculate a different range, **the inter-quartile range**. This measures the spread of the data about the median but ignores the very lowest and the very highest values. It is based, like the median, on putting the data set into ascending order, and then – as implied by the name – we split the whole data set into quarters. As an easy example we first consider a data set of eleven figures, so that we have n + 1 = 12 (which is a multiple of '4'):

2, 10, 34, 5, 7, 17, 8, 10, 30, 13, 8

First we set it in ascending order:

2, 5, 7, 8, 8, ⑩, 10, 13, 17, 30, 34

and mark the median. Since n = 11 (odd) we know that the median is the ½(n + 1)th value, that is the 6th value = '10', as shown. Working in exactly the same way, we say that the **first quartile** is the ¼(n + 1)th value, namely the 3rd value = '7'. The **third quartile** is the ¾(n + 1) th value, namely the 9th value = '17'. Here we show these three values, the first quartile, the median and the third quartile:

2, 5, 7, 8, 8, ⑩, 10, 13, 17, 30, 34

We see that the median is at mid-way, and the quartiles mark the values at the ¼ and ¾ positions. **The inter-quartile range** is '*from the first quartile to the third quartile*'. When the variable is measured at interval or ratio level then we calculate the inter-quartile range as the *difference* between the third and the first quartiles. Thus in this case:

inter-quartile range = 17 – 7 = 10

When working at interval or ratio levels of measurement we can use this method to calculate an inter-quartile range no matter how many values there are in the data set. Suppose we want the inter-quartile range of the following (already ordered) set:

2, 4, 5, 7, 8, 10, 10, 19, 34, 35

Since n = 10, we have (n + 1) = 11, so the first quartile is at the (¼ × 11)th position, that is the '2¾th' position (between the 2nd and 3rd values). We can **interpolate** here and say that the first quartile is '¾' of the way between the 2nd value, '4', and the 3rd value, '5'. The first quartile is '4¾'. Similarly, the third quartile is at the (¾ × 11)th position, that is, the '8¼ th' position. This is '¼' of the way between the 8th value, '19', and the 9th value, '34'. Thus the third quartile is '22¾'. So we have:

inter-quartile range = 22¾ – 4¾ = 18

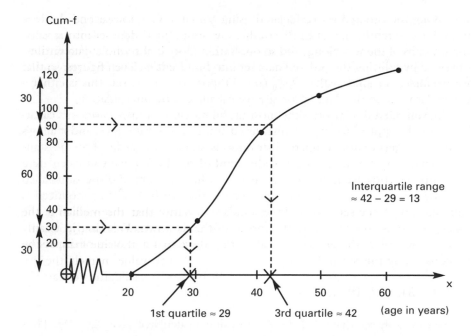

Figure 5.5   Finding an inter-quartile range graphically (like Figure 5.4 this is based on the cum-f curve of Figure 4.17)

The calculations used to obtain the inter-quartile range are simple enough for small data sets, but even then ordering is required and the interpolation can be tiresome. For large data sets the inter-quartile range is more easily estimated graphically, just as the median is. We illustrate this in Figure 5.5, the cumulative frequency curve for the nurses' ages. To find the first quartile we draw a horizontal line from the position on the y-axis which is one quarter of the way up the total frequency; where this cuts the curve shows us the value at

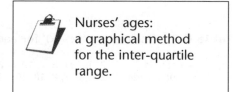

Nurses' ages: a graphical method for the inter-quartile range.

the first quartile, which is (approximately) 29 years. Starting with a horizontal line which is three-quarters of the way up the total frequency, we similarly obtain the value of the third quartile to be (approximately) 42 years. Thus the inter-quartile range of the nurses' ages is:

42 – 29 = 13

For completeness, we can here mention that just as we obtain the quartile values by splitting the whole data set into quarters, so we can obtain the **deciles** by splitting the data set into tenths. The first decile is the value one tenth of the way along the ordered set (calculated using $\frac{1}{10}(n + 1)$), the second decile is the value two tenths (i.e. one fifth) of the way along, the third decile is the value three tenths of the way along, and so on. Rather more common are **percentiles**, obtained by splitting the ordered data set into hundredths. The 55th percentile, for example, is found at the '$\frac{55}{100}(n + 1)$' position in the set: this is either a particular value in the data set or else we calculate it by interpolation.

The **standard deviation** is the most useful measure of dispersion – its calculation can be applied to any data measured at interval or ratio level and it allows us to characterise and compare distributions straightforwardly. For the standard deviation of a *sample* we use the **symbol 's'**. Before we can calculate a standard deviation we must first calculate another measure of dispersion called the **variance**, and for *sample variance* we use the **symbol 's²'** (pronounced 's squared'). Both the variance and the standard deviation are closely allied to the mean; in a sense they measure the spread of the data values about the mean.

We now look at the process for calculating these two measures of dispersion by considering this small data set:

2, 10, 34, 5, 7, 19, 4, 8, 10

We can easily see that $n = \Sigma f = 9$, and using a calculator gives $\Sigma x = 99$. Thus we have the mean:

$$\bar{x} = \frac{99}{9} = 11.$$

To see how the data values are spread about this mean value, we calculate the difference of each data value from the mean (shown in Table 5.2) and indicate the results in Figure 5.6.

Table 5.2 Calculating '$(x - \bar{x})$' for each data value

The given data is   2, 10, 34, 5, 7, 19, 4, 8, 10   (n = 9)
which we put in order 2, 4, 5, 7, 8, 10, 10, 19, 34

x	$\bar{x} = 11$	$x - \bar{x}$
2	11	$2 - 11 = -9$
4	11	-7
5	11	-6
7	11	-4
8	11	-3
10	11	-1
10	11	-1
19	11	8
34	11	23
$\Sigma x = 99$		$\Sigma(x - \bar{x}) = 0$
$\bar{x} = 11$		

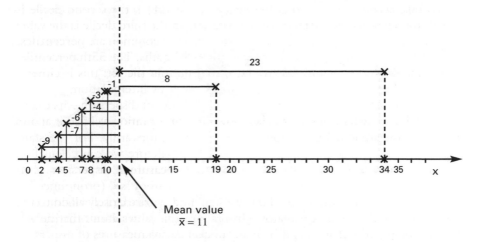

Figure 5.6 The spread of data values about the mean

What happens if we add together all these differences? That is, what happens if we calculate $\Sigma (x - \bar{x})$? The result, as indicated in Table 5.2, is zero:

$$\Sigma (x - \bar{x}) = (-9) + (-1) + 23 + (-6) + (-4) + 8 + (-7) + (-3) + (-1) = 0.$$

Fairly obviously, we will *always* get a zero answer for this – because the negative and the positive differences cancel each other out! But our measures of dispersion *must* involve the '$x - \bar{x}$' differences somehow, so we apply a trick of arithmetic here. We *square* each of the '$x - \bar{x}$' numbers (that is, we multiply each '$x - \bar{x}$' number *by itself*) and in so doing we ensure that we get a *positive* number, and it is these positive numbers we add together, giving '786', as shown in Table 5.3.

Table 5.3 Calculating the sum of squares of differences '$\Sigma(x - \bar{x})^2$'

x	$\bar{x} = 11$	$x - \bar{x}$	$(x - \bar{x})^2$
2	11	−9	$(-9)^2 = 81$
4	11	−7	49
5	11	−6	36
7	11	−4	16
8	11	−3	9
10	11	−1	1
10	11	−1	1
19	11	8	64
34	11	23	529
$\Sigma x = 99$		$\Sigma(x - \bar{x}) = 0$	$\Sigma(x - \bar{x})^2 = 786$
$\bar{x} = 11$			

To take account of the total frequency of our data set, we next divide by n = 9: this gives us the **variance** of the data set, so:

$$\text{variance} = s^2 = \frac{786}{9} = 87.33 \text{ (rounded to 2 decimal places)}$$

Finally (and again using a calculator) we find the *square root* of the variance to give us the **standard deviation**:

$$\text{standard deviation} = s = \sqrt{87.33} = 9.35 \text{ (to 2 decimal places).}$$

In Table 5.4 we summarise how we can find a standard deviation for a sample by hand – or by calculator. (In practice this is done automatically by several computer packages, and by many pocket calculators.)

Table 5.4   Steps in calculating a standard deviation of a sample of 'n' values

1.   We find *how many* values: $n = \Sigma f$,
2.   we *add up all* the values 'x': Σx,
3.   we find the *mean* of the values: $\bar{x} = \dfrac{\Sigma x}{n}$.
4.   For each value 'x' we calculate 'x – $\bar{x}$',
5.   and then *square* each one: $(x - \bar{x})^2$.
6.   We *add up* all the $(x - \bar{x})^2$: $\Sigma(x - \bar{x})^2$,
7.   and *divide* the total by n: $\dfrac{\Sigma (x - \bar{x})^2}{n}$ giving the variance, s^2.
8.   When we square root this we get the standard deviation: $$s = \sqrt{\frac{\Sigma(x - \bar{x})^2}{n}} \; .$$

The variance and the standard deviation are extremely useful measures of dispersion. They are based on *every* value in a data set and the calculations, while they may look involved, are easily followed and often automated.

5.4 Parameters and statistics

In calculating the mean or variance or standard deviation of a *sample* in the last section we were actually calculating *statistics*, in the sense of Section 3.2. We could do this because we assumed we knew exactly what all the 'n' values of the variable 'x' were. Thus the mean '$\bar{x}$', the variance 's^2' and the standard deviation 's' are all **sample statistics**.

However, when we look at a *population* (see Section 3.1) we may, or may not, know the precise number of values we are dealing with, nor the exact frequency of each one. To indicate this distinction we use different notation for the **population parameters.** For the mean of a population we use the **symbol 'μ'** (which is the Greek letter 'm', pronounced **'mew'**). For a population standard deviation we use the **symbol 'σ'** (**'sigma'** again, the lower case 's' in the Greek alphabet), and for the population variance we use the **symbol 'σ^2'** (pronounced **'sigma squared'**) (see Table 5.5).

Table 5.5 Symbols used for statistics and parameters

	Mean	*Variance*	*Standard deviation*
Sample statistic	$\bar{x}$	s^2	s
Population parameter	μ	σ^2	σ

5.5 Sufficient levels of measurement

We complete this chapter by showing in Table 5.6 the levels of measurement of the variables which are sufficient for us to calculate the key statistics of central tendency and of dispersion.

Table 5.6 The levels of measurement sufficient for calculating the key summary statistics

Statistic	*Levels of measurement*			
	Nominal	*Ordinal*	*Interval*	*Ratio*
Mode	✓	✓	✓	✓
Median		✓	✓	✓
Mean			✓	✓
Range		✓	✓	✓
Inter-quartile range		✓	✓	✓
Variance			✓	✓
Standard deviation			✓	✓

Distributions and their Curves

– *using z-scores and the standard normal curve*

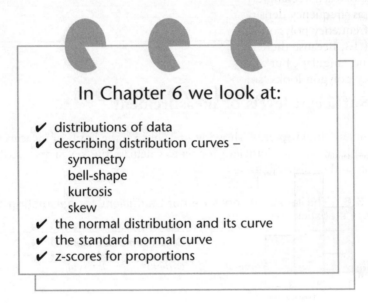

In Chapter 6 we look at:

✔ distributions of data
✔ describing distribution curves –
    symmetry
    bell-shape
    kurtosis
    skew
✔ the normal distribution and its curve
✔ the standard normal curve
✔ z-scores for proportions

Because graphs and diagrams are so important (in research papers and management reports as well as newspapers, magazines and television) we now consider how we can describe their significant features, so that we can compare them and also use them to give us statistical insights.

We know that a frequency distribution gives the overall relationship between the values taken by a variable and their frequencies (see Chapter 5), but in graphical terms a distribution describes the *overall shape of the frequency diagram*. Any frequency distribution which can be recorded on a bar chart is rather simple, so we are going to focus on frequency distributions which can be represented only by histograms. In so doing we are dealing with the majority of the real-life situations we might meet.

6.1 Frequency curves from histograms

In Section 4.2 we constructed histograms from the data collected on nurses' ages (see Figures 4.11 to 4.14). Histograms are *only* drawn when we are dealing with continuous variables, or when the quantity of data is so vast that we can validly assume that it is 'as-good-as-continuous'. Both axes measure at interval or ratio level: the x-axis always has a (continuous) scale, marked like a ruler, and the y-axis also has a ruler-like scale which we take as continuous for convenience. We remember that in a histogram the frequency is represented by the area of each rectangle (*not* its height), and the y-axis is more properly labelled as 'frequency density', 'f.d.'.

The frequency polygon shown in Figure 4.15 is based on the histogram of Figure 4.13. Because there are relatively few age-bands on the x-axis it is rather 'jerky' and 'angular', but as we increase the number of bands we can make the frequency polygon looks 'smoother'; then we call it a **frequency distribution**

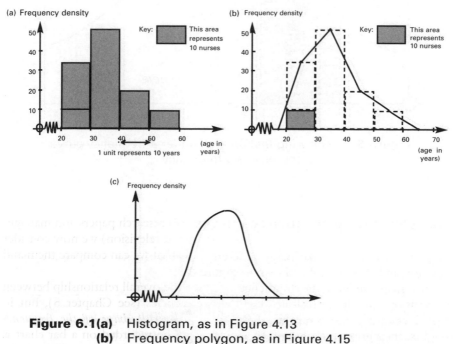

Figure 6.1(a)   Histogram, as in Figure 4.13
   (b)   Frequency polygon, as in Figure 4.15
   (c)   From a histogram to a 'smooth' frequency curve

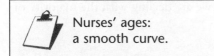

Nurses' ages:
a smooth curve.

curve or a **frequency curve** or a **distribution curve**. In Figure 6.1 we indicate the progression from a histogram to a 'smooth' frequency curve.

Every frequency curve inherits from its underlying histogram the ability to tell us about the frequencies of the values of the variable. The y-axis still measures 'frequency density' and the *area under the curve* indicates frequency. Thus the total area under a frequency curve (above the x-axis) represents the total frequency of all the values of the variable (that is, the total number of respondents in the case of our questionnaire). The area between any two vertical lines through the curve (see Figure 6.2) represents the frequency of all the values in that interval.

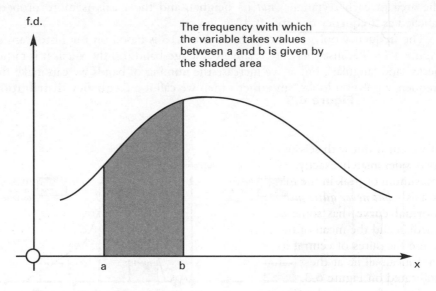

Figure 6.2   Showing that an area under a frequency curve represents a frequency

6.2 Describing frequency curves

Frequency curves can take many different possible shapes. One of the most common and most useful is shown in Figure 6.3.

This shape reflects the frequency distributions of many 'real-life' variables, including people's heights, their weights, their grip strengths and their IQs. The curve is **symmetrical**; that is,

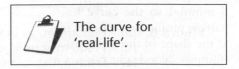

The curve for
'real-life'.

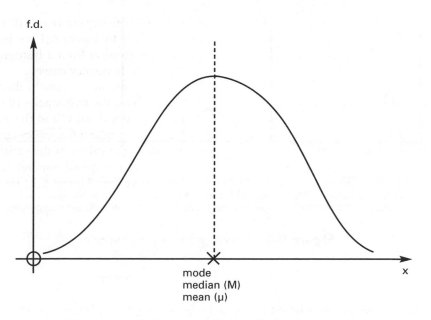

Figure 6.3   A symmetrical bell-shaped curve

if we cut it out with scissors and fold it in half along the vertical axis, then the two sides match exactly. We also see that it is **bell-shaped**, with a smooth maximum or peak in the middle and the two sides tailing off gently towards the x-axis – *but never quite meeting it.* This particular shape of curve (often called a **normal curve**) has some very useful features: if we calculate the mode, the median and the mean of the data set it represents then we find that *all three* of these measures of central location lie *at the same position.* The mode, median and mean all lie at the x-value where the curve reaches its peak – this point is indicated on Figure 6.3.

Other frequency distributions can be symmetrical like the one in Figure 6.3 but might differ in the extent to which the central peak is taller or more flattened. This quality of 'peakedness' is known as **kurtosis**, and in Figure 6.4 we show three symmetrical curves with different degrees of kurtosis.

Figure 6.4(a) shows a **leptokurtic** curve, with a very pronounced peak. An example of this shape is in the frequency distribution of the (fasting) blood glucose levels throughout a *healthy* population: the overall range of the glucose levels is between 4 and 8 mmol/l so the curve has quite a narrow profile. In contrast, if we look at the shape of the distribution of the (fasting) blood glucose levels in a

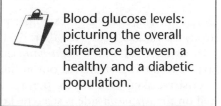

Blood glucose levels: picturing the overall difference between a healthy and a diabetic population.

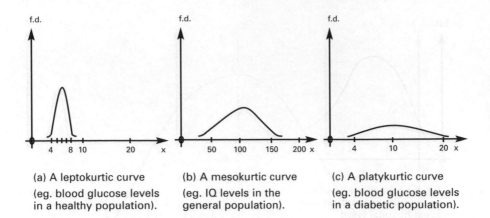

(a) A leptokurtic curve
(eg. blood glucose levels
in a healthy population).

(b) A mesokurtic curve
(eg. IQ levels in the
general population).

(c) A platykurtic curve
(eg. blood glucose levels
in a diabetic population).

Figure 6.4   Curves with varying kurtosis

diabetic population (where the overall range of the glucose levels is from below 4 mmol/l to maybe more than 20 mmol/l) the values are well spread out so the curve appears very broad and rather flattened: this is called a **platykurtic** curve (see Figure 6.4(c)). In between these two shapes we have the normal curve which is **mesokurtic** (Figure 6.4(b), neither 'extra' narrow nor 'extra' broad; an example of this shape is in the distribution of the Intelligence Quotients (IQs) of the general population. (These prefixes: **lepto**, **meso**- and **platy**-, just mean 'slender', 'middling' and 'broad' respectively.)

The kurtosis of a distribution can be measured and expressed as a single number, but we shall not deal with these calculations. It turns out that a mesokurtic curve has 'zero kurtosis'. When a curve is leptokurtic it has positive kurtosis, and the 'more peaked' it is, the higher the number. A platykurtic curve has a negative kurtosis value.

Sometimes the curve of a frequency distribution is not symmetrical. An instance of this is the curve of the distribution of lengths of inpatient stay in an acute hospital ward. Here, increasing numbers of patients are discharged after 1, 2 or 3 days and most are discharged on days 4 or 5; this leaves declining numbers to be discharged daily thereafter. This is an example where the curve is slightly asymmetric and one of its 'tails' stretches out further from the middle than the other: we have a **skewed** distribution. In this particular case the tail on the *right-hand* side stretches out much further along the x-axis; because it is stretched out in the direction of the *positive* x-axis it is called a **positive skew** (see Figure 6.5(a)). A curve with a **negative skew**, where the tail on the *left-hand* side is stretched out further along the x-axis in the *negative*

Picturing lengths of inpatient stay.

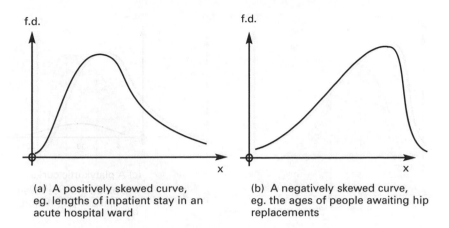

(a) A positively skewed curve,
eg. lengths of inpatient stay in an
acute hospital ward

(b) A negatively skewed curve,
eg. the ages of people awaiting hip
replacements

Figure 6.5   Curves with varying skew

direction, is shown in Figure 6.5(b). A negative skew occurs in the distribution of the ages of people awaiting hip replacements: relatively few young people need hip replacements but the numbers increase with age, then very few replacements are offered to very old people.

Picturing the ages of those awaiting hip replacements.

When dealing with a skewed curve we see that the mode and the median of the distribution are never the same. The mode remains at the position corresponding to the maximum point on the curve but the median (M) is 'pulled sideways' by the increased number of values in one direction. Half of the total number of values of the variable (that is, half of the total frequency) are less than the median and half are greater than the median; because of this the median moves to a position where the *area* under the curve to the left of it is equal to the *area* under the curve to the right of it. As we see in Figure 6.6, in a positively skewed distribution the median is greater than the mode, but if the distribution is negatively skewed then the median is less than the mode.

Types of curves that are completely unsymmetric can also exhibit skewness. In Figure 6.7 we show two **J-curves** where the frequencies are 'piled high' at just one end of the x-axis and tail off at the other. Figure 6.7(a) shows a **positively skewed J-curve** which could arise from the distribution of the time past their 'estimated due date' that overdue pregnant women wait to give birth (the majority frequencies are for one or two days, then the numbers

Picturing times waiting to give birth.

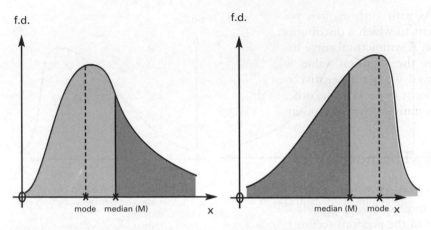

mode median (M)   median (M)   mode

In a positively skewed distribution,
median > mode

In a negatively skewed distribution,
median < mode

Figure 6.6   The relationships between means and medians on skewed curves; the areas either side of the median line are equal

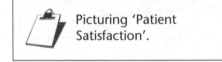

Picturing 'Patient Satisfaction'.

rapidly tail-off). A different situation arises if we draw a curve for 'Patient Satisfaction' (rated on a 1–10 scale with '10' indicating high satisfaction). It is known that the majority of patients are satisfied with the care they receive and very few give returns at the lower end of the scale. Figure 6.7(b) shows an example of this shape of curve; it is a **negatively skewed J-curve**.

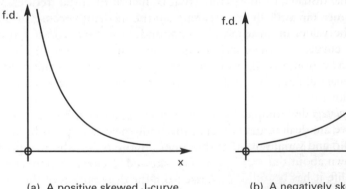

(a) A positive skewed J-curve,
eg. time past EDD that overdue
pregnant women wait

(b) A negatively skewed J-curve,
eg. 'Patient Satisfaction'

Figure 6.7   J-curves

As with kurtosis, it is possible to calculate a single number to reflect the extent to which a distribution is skewed – but we shall not go into the details here. A symmetrical curve has 'zero skewness'; when a curve is positively skewed then the skewness value is a positive number and when it is negatively skewed we get a negative number. The greater the degree of 'piling up' of values at one end or the other of the x-axis, then the greater the *size* of the skewness number (whether positive or negative).

6.3 The normal distribution

The **normal distribution**, applied to a *population*, is the name given to one of the most common real-life distributions (which we began to introduce at the start of the previous section). It occurs in a wide variety of situations, especially in natural populations when we are dealing with physical or practical attributes from large samples of living organisms (plants, animals or humans). Human characteristics are often determined by many different factors, and when measured over populations we find they are normally distributed, for example temperature, weight, lung

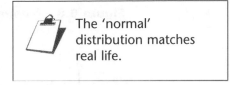

The 'normal' distribution matches real life.

volume, vital capacity and IQs. The key features of this distribution are that all the values cluster around a single central location, there are approximately as many values above this central location as there are below it and, the further we get from the central location, the fewer values there are. When these features are translated into graphical terms we see that the distribution curve is mesokurtic with a single smooth peak, is symmetric about a line through that maximum and it 'tails away' as it approaches the x-axis on either side. In fact the distribution curve for the normal distribution is precisely the symmetrical, bell-shaped curve that we saw in Figure 6.3 and the area beneath the curve represents the total frequency of all the values of the variable. In Figure 6.8 we show this shape again: the **normal curve**.

As mentioned in Section 6.2, on this bell-shaped normal curve the mode, the median and the mean all have the same value, $M = \mu$, which corresponds with the maximum point on the curve. In addition, any normal distribution of a population is *completely* determined by the values of its mean and its standard deviation. When we are dealing with such a normal distribution, with mean μ, standard deviation σ and variance σ^2, we commonly write it as $N(\mu, \sigma^2)$. There is a great deal known about this distribution and its curve: because it occurs so frequently in real life it has been much studied and its properties are used for many purposes.

Since normal curves can arise in many situations, referring to different variables in different populations, the graphs can *appear* to be different (see Figure 6.9).

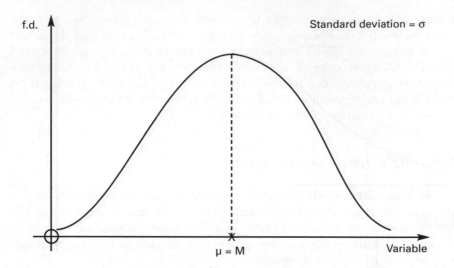

Figure 6.8   A normal curve N(μ, σ^2)

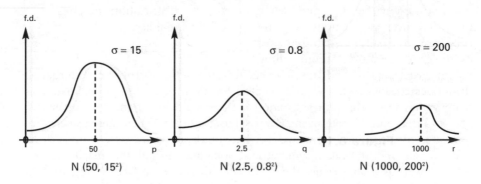

Figure 6.9   Normal curves at different scales

We use a technique called **standardising** to reduce them all to the same shape and scale so that we can analyse them. Once we have standardised a normal curve then its mean is 'zero', its standard deviation is 'one' and the total area under the curve is also 'one'.

On a **standard normal curve** there is a special relationship between the horizontal scale and the standard deviation. Suppose we mark off the horizontal scale, from the origin, not just in numbers but in *multiples of the standard deviation,* and then draw vertical lines at the -3σ, -2σ, -1σ, $+1\sigma$, $+2\sigma$, and 3σ marks, as shown in Figure 6.10(a). We see that virtually the whole area under the standard normal curve lies between the lines at -3σ and $+3\sigma$ (this is actually 99.5% of the area).

In the same way the area lying between each pair of the lines is a known

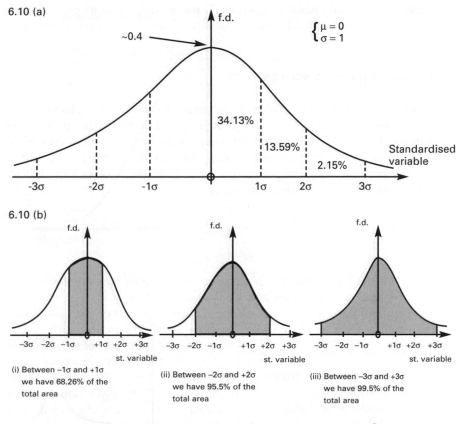

Figure 6.10 The standard normal curve N(0,1²)

percentage or proportion of the whole area: the section between 'zero' (the mean) and 'plus one standard deviation' contains 34.13% of the area; the section between one and two standard deviations above the mean contains 13.59% of the whole area; and between two and three standard deviations above the mean we have 2.15% of the whole area. The curve is symmetrical so the sections on the negative side of the axis contain matching percentages of the total area. Thus between plus and minus one standard deviation we have 68.26% of the area, between plus and minus two standard deviations we have 95.5% of the area, and between plus and minus three standard deviations we have 99.5% of the area (see Figure 6.10(b)). We can obtain these areas and many more, as percentages or proportions, from the Table in Appendix 5(b). These figures are very useful because, once we know the percentage/proportion of area we have (between two vertical lines) we also know the percentage/proportion of the total frequency we are dealing with (between two given values of the variable). In addition, since probability and relative frequency are closely connected as we shall discuss in Chapter 7, we are often able to use standard-ised normal curves to calculate the probability of particular events occurring.

6.4　Standardised scores

How do we *standardise* a normal curve, so that we can obtain results using the Table in Appendix 5(b)? The method is simple. For each relevant value of the variable, x, we calculate its **standard score**, or **z-score**, using the values of the population mean, μ, and the population standard deviation, σ. We obtain the z-score by subtracting the population mean from the value of x then divid-ing by the (population) standard deviation:

$$z = \frac{x - \mu}{\sigma}$$

Then the standardised curve has its mean at 'zero' and its horizontal axis (now called the *z-axis*) is scaled in multiples of the standard deviation.

As an example, we now use the above ideas to explore how we would esti-mate quantities for a purchase order. Suppose we are responsible for purchas-ing pairs of sterile gloves to be used by the 25,000 female nursing staff employed by a Regional Health Authority. The gloves come in five sizes, extra-small (XS), small (S), Medium (M), large (L) and extra-large (XL); we must decide how many pairs of each size to order.

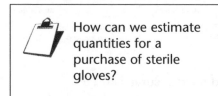

How can we estimate quantities for a purchase of sterile gloves?

We start by obtaining the measurements of nurses' hand sizes from a random sample of 1250 female nurses (the measurements are in centimetres, to the nearest 0.1 cm, measured around the knuckles of the dominant hand). We use the calculations already described in Sections 5.2 and 5.3 to find the mean, $\bar{x}$, and the standard deviation, s, of these measurements. We can assume that the population, that is *all* nurses' hand sizes, is normally distributed and since our sample is *very large* we shall take it (in this case, but not always! – see Chapters 8 and 9) that the values of $\bar{x}$ and s give us good approximations for μ and σ. Suppose we find that:

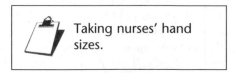

Taking nurses' hand sizes.

$$\bar{x} = 18.1 \text{ (cm)} \quad \text{so we take } \mu = 18.1 \text{ (cm)}$$
$$\text{and} \quad s = 2.1 \text{ (cm)} \quad \text{so we take } \sigma = 2.1 \text{ (cm)}$$

We can calculate the z-score for the case when the variable takes the value x = 19.6 cm (say):

$$z = \frac{x - \mu}{\sigma} = \frac{19.6 - 18.1}{2.1} = \frac{1.5}{2.1} = 0.71 \text{ (to 2 decimal places)}$$

This indicates that an original value of x = 19.6 cm corresponds to the point on the standardised normal curve where z = 0.71, that is 0.71 of a standard deviation to the right of the mean (see Figure 6.11).

Before returning to our example on purchasing gloves, we practice using the information in Figure 6.11, together with the Table in Appendix 5(b), to find out how many nurses in our sample have different hand measurements. Of course these results (for the sample) can be verified directly against the numbers we have collected.

> How many nurses have the different hand sizes?

We start by finding how many there are with hand sizes bigger than 19.6 cm (which we calculated has the z-score of z = 0.71). In Table 6.1 we show part of the Table from Appendix 5(b); it has eleven columns. The first column, headed by 'z', contains the 'first decimal place' of our z-score. If our z-score were '0.7 exactly' then (since 0.7 is the same as 0.70) we would read off the four-digit decimal number alongside the '0.7' in the second column, headed by '0'; this is '0.2420'. But since our z-score is '0.71', correct to two decimal places, we move along this row and read off the four-digit decimal number in the column headed by '1'; this is '0.2389'. (Similarly, if the z-score is '0.78', we move along the '0.7' row until we are in the column headed '8' and read off the four-digit decimal number there; namely '0.2177'.) Since these

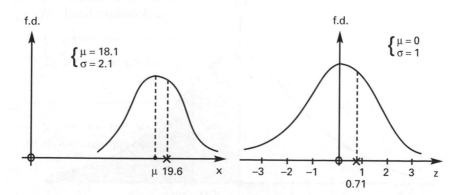

Figure 6.11 Comparing a normal curve with the standardised normal curve

Table 6.1 Part of the table of the standard normal distribution (taken from Appendix 5(b))

	0	1	2	3	4	5	6	7	8	9
0.0	0.5000	0.4960	0.4920	0.4880	0.4840	0.4801	0.4761	0.4721	0.4681	0.4641
0.1	0.4602	0.4562	0.4522	0.4483	0.4443	0.4404	0.4364	0.4325	0.4286	0.4247
0.2	0.4207	0.4168	0.4129	0.4090	0.4052	0.4013	0.3974	0.3936	0.3897	0.3859
0.3	0.3821	0.3783	0.3745	0.3707	0.3669	0.3632	0.3594	0.3557	0.3520	0.3483
0.4	0.3446	0.3409	0.3372	0.3336	0.3300	0.3264	0.3228	0.3192	0.3156	0.3121
0.5	0.3085	0.3050	0.3015	0.2981	0.2946	0.2912	0.2877	0.2843	0.2810	0.2776
0.6	0.2743	0.2709	0.2676	0.2643	0.2611	0.2578	0.2546	0.2514	0.2483	0.2451
0.7	0.2420	0.2389	0.2358	0.2327	0.2296	0.2266	0.2236	0.2206	0.2177	0.2148
0.8	0.2119	0.2090	0.2061	0.2033	0.2005	0.1977	0.1949	0.1922	0.1894	0.1867
0.9	0.1841	0.1814	0.1788	0.1762	0.1736	0.1711	0.1685	0.1660	0.1635	0.1611
1.0	0.1587	0.1562	0.1539	0.1515	0.1492	0.1469	0.1446	0.1423	0.1401	0.1379
1.1	0.1357	0.1335	0.1314	0.1292	0.1271	0.1251	0.1230	0.1210	0.1190	0.1170

Tables are 'right-hand tail' tables, these four-digit decimal numbers tell us the proportion of the whole area which lies *to the right* of a vertical line through the z-score in question.

For the hand measurement 'x = 19.6' the z-score is 'z = 0.71' and so the proportion of area to the right, shown shaded in Figure 6.12, is given by the number '0.2389': Since the proportion of area under this curve corresponds with the proportion of the total frequency (1250 in this case) we have:

$$0.2389 \times 1250 = 299 \text{ (approx)}$$

and so approximately 299 nurses in our sample have hand sizes bigger than 19.6 cm.

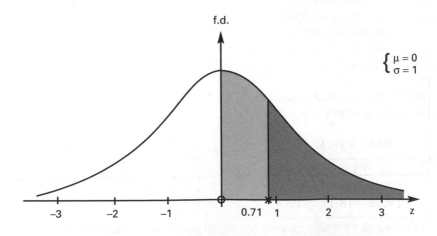

Figure 6.12 The proportion of area to the right of z = 0.71

We can also find the expected number of nurses in the sample with hand sizes *smaller* than 19.6 cm – we use simple subtraction:

$$1250 - 299 = 951$$

and so there are 951 of them.

If we want the number of nurses in the sample whose hand size is greater than the mean but less than 19.6 cm, we recognise that because of the symmetry of the curve the areas on each side are equal, and each represents precisely half the total frequency, that is half of 1250, namely 625. The frequency we require is that represented by the pale grey area in Figure 6.12, which is

$$625 - 299 = 326.$$

Thus 326 nurses in our sample have hand sizes between 18.1 cm and 19.6 cm.

We must be very careful when we are using a normal curve to answer questions about the frequency of a *single value*, for example 'How many nurses in the sample have a hand size of *exactly 19.6 cm?*' This is because all frequencies in a normal distribution are represented by *areas* under the normal curve, and a single straight line (marking x = 19.6 cm) has no thickness and so cannot, by itself, indicate an area (see Figure 6.13). We get around this by recognising that

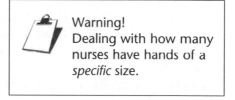

Warning!
Dealing with how many nurses have hands of a *specific* size.

since 'hand size' is a continuous variable, the measurement x = 19.6 cm actually refers to a whole set of measurements: all of the measurements from 19.55 cm up to (but not including) 19.65 cm would 'round' to the same 19.6 cm, accurate to one place of decimals (we met this idea in Section 4.1). For this set of measurements that we would record as '19.6 cm' the class boundaries are 19.55 cm and 19.65 cm, and we draw vertical lines though these to identify the appropriate section of area under the curve. In Figure 6.13 we see this area shaded.

To find the required frequency we first calculate (correct to two places of decimals) the z-scores of x_A = 19.55 and x_B = 19.65 respectively:

$$z_A = \frac{19.55 - 18.1}{2.1} = \frac{1.45}{2.1} = 0.69$$

$$z_B = \frac{19.65 - 18.1}{2.1} = \frac{1.55}{2.1} = 0.74$$

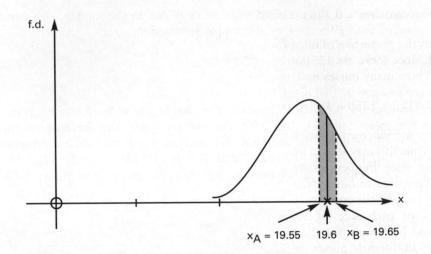

Figure 6.13   The area from which we find the frequency of 'x = 19.6'

From Table 6.1 (or Appendix 5(b)) we see that the proportion of area to the right of the z-score 'z_A = 0.69' is '0.2451', and the proportion of area to the right of the z-score 'z_B = 0.74' is '0.2296'; we illustrate these proportions in Figure 6.14.

To find the proportion of area within the required section we subtract these values:

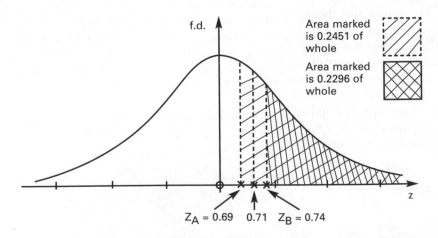

Figure 6.14   The section of area about the value 'z = 0.71'
(the z-score of 'x = 19.6')

required area = 0.2451 − 0.2296 = 0.0155

Thus the *proportion* of nurses who give their hand size as '19.6 cm' is '0.0155', and, since there are 1250 nurses in the sample, we multiply these numbers to find how many nurses have this hand size:

0.0155 × 1250 = 19 (rounded to the nearest whole number)

There are nineteen nurses with hand size 19.6 cm.

While this may seem a long-winded way to calculate the frequency of a single value, since 'frequencies are represented by areas' there is really no alternative!

Returning to our purchasing exercise: we wish to use the information from our sample to estimate how many pairs of each size of sterile glove should be bought for the population of 25,000 female nurses employed by a Regional Health Authority. The measurements of the five sizes of gloves are shown in Table 6.2.

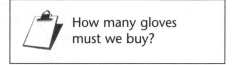 How many gloves must we buy?

Table 6.2 Glove sizes and hand sizes

Glove size	Knuckle circumference
XS (extra small	less than 16 cm
S (small)	16 cm but less than 17.5 cm
M (medium)	17.5 cm but less than 18.5 cm
L (large)	18.5 cm but less than 19.5 cm
XL (extra large)	19 cm or more

We assume that the population of hand sizes is normally distributed and we have assumed, from our (very large) sample of 1250 nurses, that the mean of this distribution is $\mu = 18.1$ cm and the standard deviation is $\sigma = 2.1$ cm. To find the proportions of the population requiring the different glove sizes we must find the proportions of area (under the normal curve) between the vertical lines which correspond to the boundaries between glove sizes. These are shown in Table 6.3 and in Figure 6.15.

We calculate the z-scores for these boundary values and show them on the standard normal curve (see Figure 6.16):

$$z_1 = \frac{16 - 18.1}{2.1} = \frac{-2.1}{2.1} = -1$$

$$z_2 = \frac{17.5 - 18.1}{2.1} = \frac{-0.6}{2.1} = -0.29$$

Table 6.3   The boundaries between glove sizes

Glove size	Knuckle circumference	Lower boundary (cm)	Upper boundary (cm)
XS (extra small)	less than 16 cm	–	16
S (small)	16 cm but less than 17.5 cm	16	17.5
M (medium)	17.5 cm but less than 28.5 cm	17.5	18.5
L (large)	18.5 cm but less than 29.5 cm	18.5	19.5
XL (extra large)	19.5 cm or more	19.5	–

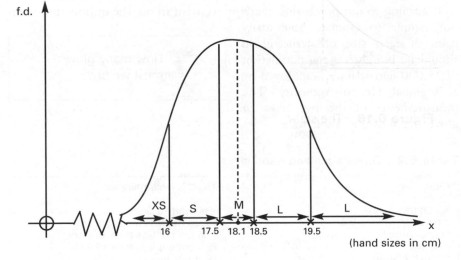

Figure 6.15   Normal curve of hand sizes showing the boundaries for glove sizes

$$z_3 = \frac{18.5 - 18.1}{2.1} = \frac{0.4}{2.1} = 0.19$$

$$z_4 = \frac{19.5 - 18.1}{2.1} = \frac{1.4}{2.1} = 0.67$$

(all correct to 2 places of decimals)

Using now the more complete Table in Appendix 5(b), we use subtraction to find the proportion of areas between these z-scores.

From the Table, the proportion of area *to the right* of z_4 is '0.2514'. The proportion of area to the right of z_3 is '0.4247', so subtracting the '0.2514' gives the proportion of area *between* z_3 and z_4 to be '0.1733' (see Figure

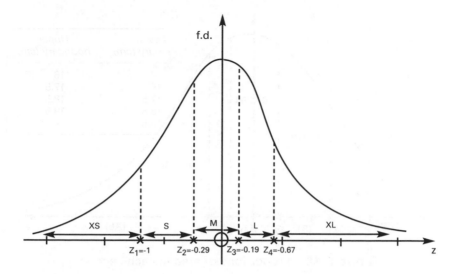

Figure 6.16 The standard normal curve for hand sizes, showing boundaries for glove sizes

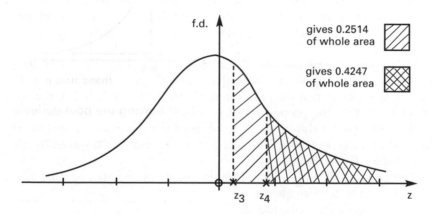

Figure 6.17 The process of subtracting areas

6.17, where the area to the right of z_4 is hatched one way and that to the right of z_3 is hatched the other: we obviously require the *difference* between these). Figure 6.18 shows the proportions of the area between z_3 and z_4 and to the right of z_4.

Since z_1 and z_2 have *negative values*, we now proceed with some care. First we consider z_1: if we start by ignoring the minus sign we can look at the number in the Table which corresponds to '$z = 1$' – this number is '0.1587'. However, because z_1 is *negative* this number gives the proportion of area *to the*

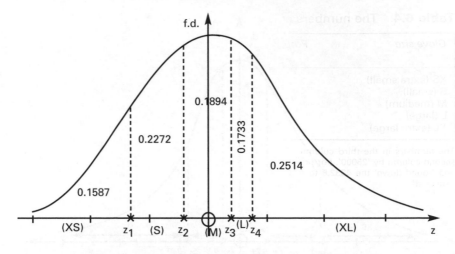

Figure 6.18 Proportions of area in each section

left of z_1 (as shown in Figure 6.18). Similarly, ignoring the minus sign on z_2, the number we obtain from the Table for '$z = 0.29$' is '0.3859', which is the proportion of area *to the left* of z_2. So subtracting '0.1587' from '0.3859' gives the number '0.2272' which is the proportion of area between z_1 and z_2 (see Figure 6.18).

Finally we want the proportion of area between z_2 and z_3. We obtain this by remembering that the whole area beneath a standardised normal curve is '1'. To the left of z_2 we know that the proportion of area is '0.3859', and to the right of z_3 we know that the proportion of area is '0.4247'; we add these to get '0.8106', and subtract this from '1' to obtain the proportion of area 'in the middle'. Thus the proportion of the area between z_2 and z_3 is '$1 - 0.8106$', that is '0.1894' (see Figure 6.18).

The proportions of these areas under the graph are exactly the same as the proportions of the total frequency of the whole population considered. Thus, to find the numbers of pairs of gloves to be purchased in each of the five sizes, we multiply the proportions we have calculated by the total frequency, 25,000. We summarise these results in Table 6.4. These figures give us an informed estimate on which to base the purchase order of the sterile gloves.

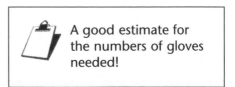

A good estimate for the numbers of gloves needed!

Table 6.4   The numbers of pairs of gloves to be purchased

Glove size	Proportion of area	Numbers of pairs of gloves to be purchased
XS (extra small)	0.1587	3967.5
S (small)	0.2272	5680
M (medium)	0.1894	4735
L (large)	0.1733	4332.5
XL (extra large)	0.2514	6285

The numbers in the third column are obtained by multiplying the corresponding numbers in the second column by '25000'. For practical purposes we could decide to 'round up' the 3967.5 to 3968, and 'round down' the 4332.5 to 4332 (or vice versa). The third column *does* add up to 25000, as expected!

Is it Likely?

– using ideas of probability and significance testing

7

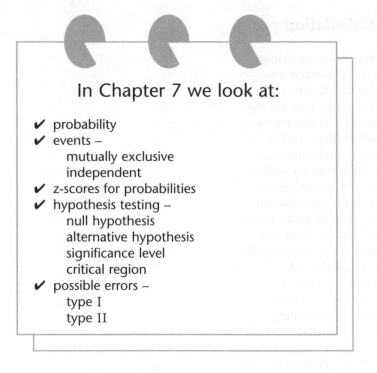

In Chapter 7 we look at:

✔ probability
✔ events –
  mutually exclusive
  independent
✔ z-scores for probabilities
✔ hypothesis testing –
  null hypothesis
  alternative hypothesis
  significance level
  critical region
✔ possible errors –
  type I
  type II

Words like 'probable', 'likely' and 'sure' are very common in most people's vocabulary; they indicate us trying to get to grips with **chance** and **uncertainty**. For example: 'It is *probable* that this patient can go home tomorrow', or '*How sure* are we that this combination of drugs will be more effective than that single drug?', or 'What is the *probability* that it will rain today?', or 'It is *likely* that this treatment will improve the patient's mobility', or 'Can we say *how certain* we are that no intervention is necessary?'.

The **descriptive statistics** we have looked at so far lead us to ways of quantifying our ideas of probability which, in turn, lead us to the methods of **inferential statistics** that we shall be exploring in the rest of this book. While it can be a straightforward matter to record and analyse just how many patients get better after a clinical trial, it is clearly essential to determine (with an agreed level of confidence) whether in some cases the patient recovery might be a chance happening, *probably not* influenced by the experimental treatment. The understanding of how we regard hypothetical events (or events in the future) and estimate their likelihood, is the key to our developing these essential tools for judging between 'probable' and 'improbable' events.

7.1 Calculating probability

Most **events** or **outcomes** (when a particular variable takes specific values) cannot be predicted completely accurately – there is always some level of uncertainty. Despite this, we intuitively know that some events are 'more probable' and some are 'less probable' and it is useful to be able to make comparisons. There are two main approaches to understanding and calculating **probability**, and it is by *calculating probabilities* that we can make *informed* judgements and decisions.

The first way to understand probability follows a **classical approach**. In this, any 'event' is considered as the one that 'actually happens' from among all the possible outcomes which *might* have happened. To apply this method we need to know *precise numbers* for 'how many ways this event can happen' and for 'how many possible outcomes there are altogether'. The easiest examples of this approach come from rather artificial (non-clinical) fields: coin tossing, dice throwing, card dealing and similar gambling activities!

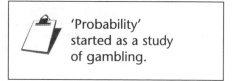
'Probability' started as a study of gambling.

As a simple example we consider an experiment where we toss four unbiased (that is, 'fair') coins simultaneously: we want to know the probability that the event 'precisely two Heads show' arises. In how many ways can this happen? and how many possible outcomes are there altogether? These issues can be explored using a table: Table 7.1 shows the results for each coin ('H' for 'Head' and 'T' for 'Tail') in *all the possible outcomes* for the experiment. We see that there are *sixteen possible* outcomes, and in *just six* of the outcomes we have 'precisely two Heads show'.

By this way of calculating probability we have:

Table 7.1   All possible outcomes when tossing four coins

Outcome	Coin 1	Coin 2	Coin 3	Coin 4	Number of heads
1	H	H	H	H	4
2	H	H	H	T	3
3	H	H	T	H	3
4	H	T	H	H	3
5	T	H	H	H	3
6	H	H	T	T	2
7	H	T	H	T	2
8	T	H	H	T	2
9	H	T	T	H	2
10	T	H	T	H	2
11	T	T	H	H	2
12	H	T	T	T	1
13	T	H	T	T	1
14	T	T	H	T	1
15	T	T	T	H	1
16	T	T	T	T	0

$$\text{probability of event} = \frac{number\ of\ ways\ event\ occurs}{total\ number\ of\ possible\ outcomes}$$

which can be written using 'shorthand' as

$$p(event) = \frac{number\ of\ ways\ event\ occurs}{total\ number\ of\ possible\ outcomes}$$

Thus in the coin tossing case we have:

$$p(\text{precisely 2 Heads show}) = \frac{number\ of\ ways\ '2\ Heads'\ occurs}{total\ number\ of\ possible\ outcomes}$$

$$= \frac{6}{16} = \frac{3}{8} = 0.375$$

The second way in which probabilities can be understood and measured, called the **empirical approach**, relates more to our experience of real life. By repeated trials of 'experiments' over extended periods, we often get 'a feel' for the **relative frequency** of any given event occurring, where, as in Section 4.1:

$$\text{relative frequency} = \frac{frequency\ of\ the\ event}{total\ frequency}$$

There are many situations where, *in the long term*, relative frequencies 'settle down' to a consistent figure which we feel is 'correct'. The correctness of this 'feel' can be validated, as required, by further trials. An example of this is the relative frequency with which a girl baby is born, compared with all the births in a Trust's area. Over a long enough time span, we find (to a good approximation):

> Roughly half of all babies born are girls (as expected!).

$$\text{relative frequency} = \frac{\textit{frequency of girl baby births}}{\textit{total frequency of all births}} = \frac{1}{2}$$

When we have a value for the long term *relative frequency* of a particular event, then we interpret that figure as the *probability* of that event. Thus, in the absence of interventions, for any conception:

$$p(\text{a baby is a girl}) = \frac{1}{2}$$

In general, when the trends are clear, we can always interpret that 'relative frequency in the past' is the same as 'probability for the present or future'.

When we calculate the probability of an event, we get the *same result* whether we employ the classical or the empirical method. We can verify this in a simple case where either method can be used: consider what happens when we toss a single unbiased coin. How do we 'know' that the probability of getting 'a Head' is ½? By the classical method we reason that there is *just one* way to achieve the desired event, 'a Head', out of *two possible outcomes*, 'a Head' or 'a Tail'. Thus:

$$p(\text{a Head}) = \frac{\textit{number of ways 'a Head' occurs}}{\textit{total number of possible outcomes}} = \frac{1}{2}$$

Alternatively we might toss the coin repeatedly (perhaps a hundred times or more) recording 'Head' or 'Tail' each time, and apply empirical reasoning. After each toss we calculate the relative frequency of Heads up to that point. As the sequence of tosses progresses we see that the numbers for the relative frequency of Heads approach closer and closer to the value ½. Whichever method is used, the probability of 'a Head' is the same: ½. (By similar methods, the probability of 'a Tail' is identical: p(a Tail) = p(a Head) = ½.)

Whichever method is used, the probability of any event is always calculated to be a positive number between zero and '1'. As in the 'tossing four coins' example above, we can leave it as a *fraction*, eg. '⅜', or we can convert it to *decimal* notation, as here '0.375'. It is also quite common to record probabilities as *percentages*, in this case it would be '37.5%'. These three results are all equivalent.

There are two 'special' values of probabilities. If an event is *absolutely certain* then its probability is 'one', thus:

> The extreme probabilities: 'dead certs' and 'absolutely impossible'.

p ('dead cert') = 1

Because of this, without further calculation we have

p (a normally healthy man has a spine) = 1
p (a tossed coin will fall back to the ground) = 1
p (each woman now alive will die) = 1

On the other hand, if an event is *absolutely impossible* then its probability is 'zero', thus:

p ('an impossibility') = 0

Thus we immediately know that

p (a normally healthy man has green blood) = 0
p (a tossed coin will remain suspended in mid-air) = 0
p (elephants and salmon can mate naturally) = 0

We can envisage extreme situations where we suppose the probabilities are *very close* to 'one' or 'zero'. That a woman aged 105 will give birth to a baby in the next twenty years has an *extremely small probability* (near to 'zero') – but we cannot say definitely that the probability *is* 'zero'. That the average number of years that transplant patients survive will continue to rise has a *very high probability* (near to 'one'), and yet we cannot state categorically that the probability *is* 'one'. All probabilities are values between 'zero' (for impossibilities) and 'one' (for dead certs), but most of them take the fractional values in-between 'zero' and 'one'.

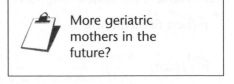

> More geriatric mothers in the future?

> Will transplant patients survive a natural lifespan?

7.2 Combining probabilities

When and how is it possible to combine probabilities? If a family already has five daughters, what is the probability that the sixth child is also a daughter? If we know the overall probabilities that anyone in our area is a wheelchair user or is a vegetarian, what is the probability that the next person to visit the clinic is both a wheelchair user and a vegetarian? Suppose we want the probability that a female patient is potentially capable of child-bearing: how can we calculate the probability that a woman is either pregnant or infertile? If we know the probability of a hereditary condition affecting one child in a family, what is the probability that a second or third child is affected? If the overall probability of an allergic reaction to a particular drug is known, what is the probability of a woman being allergic? or a teenager? or a baby? The answers to these questions depend crucially on the nature of the events themselves and how they are connected. We first look at the two basic ways in which events can be related and we shall return to discuss these particular questions later in this section.

We say that two events are **mutually exclusive** if there is no possible way that they can both happen (at the same time). Thus the events 'the next baby boy born in this delivery suite weighs below 3 kg' and 'the next baby boy born in this delivery suite weighs over 4 kg' are mutually exclusive: *either* one event may happen *or* the other (or maybe neither) – but they can *not both* happen. For *mutually exclusive* events we can *add* the indi-

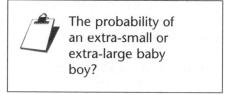

The probability of an extra-small or extra-large baby boy?

vidual probabilities to get the probability of **either/or**. Thus if we know (approximately):

p (next full-term baby boy born weighs below 3 kg) = 0.09

and

p (next full-term baby boy born weighs over 4 kg) = 0.25

we can combine these and say

p (next full-term baby boy born weighs *either* less than 3 kg *or* more than 4 kg) = 0.09 + 0.25 = 0.34.

Returning to our experiment of tossing a single unbiased coin: the two possible events, 'a Head' and 'a Tail', are mutually exclusive – they cannot both happen at the same time. We already know that:

$$p \text{ (a Head)} = p \text{ (a Tail)} = \frac{1}{2}$$

so we can combine these and say

$$p \text{ (\textit{either} a Head \textit{or} a Tail)} = \frac{1}{2} + \frac{1}{2} = 1$$

This completely fits with our experience because, on tossing a coin, it is a 'dead cert' that we get the event of *either* a Head *or* a Tail (no other possibility exists).

Two events are **independent** if the occurrence of one happening has no effect whatsoever on whether the other happens or not. We can easily see that the events 'the patient was a stroke victim' and 'the patient wore brown slippers' are quite independent and unconnected. On the other hand we would not say that 'the patient was in the geriatric ward' and 'the patient had grey hair' are independent events, since age and hair colour are often related. When we know the probabilities of individual *independent* events, then we can combine them by *multiplication* to determine the probability of **both/and**. Thus if we know:

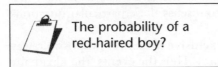

The probability of a red-haired boy?

$$p \text{ (the child is a girl)} = 0.5$$

and also:

$$p \text{ (the child has red hair)} = 0.03 \text{ (say)}$$

then, since these events are independent we can calculate:

$$p \text{ (the child is \textit{both} a girl \textit{and} she has red hair)} = 0.5 \times 0.03 = 0.015$$

In the context of coin tossing experiments, we can consider what happens when we toss an unbiased coin twice over: the result of the first toss has no influence at all on the result of the second toss – they are independent events. We use this to calculate the probability of the event 'first a Head, then a Tail'. Since we know that:

$$p \text{ (a Head)} = p \text{ (a Tail)} = 0.5$$

we have:

$$p \text{ (a Head \textit{and} then a Tail)} = 0.5 \times 0.5 = 0.25$$

If we toss four unbiased coins simultaneously, then each shows an event of 'a Head' or 'a Tail' that is completely independent of all of the others, so we can use this to calculate the probability of getting the combined event 'four Tails'. We know that:

p (a Tail) = 0.5

and so

p (a Tail *and* a Tail *and* a Tail *and* a Tail) = $0.5 \times 0.5 \times 0.5 \times 0.5 = 0.0625$
(with a calculator)

We see that this answer matches the result we would get using Table 7.1:

$$p \text{ (4 Tails)} = \frac{number\ of\ ways\ `4\ Tails'\ occurs}{total\ number\ of\ possible\ outcomes}$$

$$= \frac{1}{16} = 0.0625$$

(We note that mutually exclusive events, that can only occur in the absence of the other, are by that fact logically connected to each other: mutually exclusive events are *never* independent of each other.)

We now return to the questions with which we began this section.

If a family already has five daughters, what is the probability that the sixth child is also a daughter? As we already know:

What chance an 'all girls' family?

p (a baby is a boy) = p (a baby is a girl) = 0.5

but the gender of each new baby is an independent event, not influenced by any other event. Thus the probability that a family with five children already has five daughters is rather small, shown by multiplying the probabilities together:

p (daughter 1 *and* daughter 2 *and* daughter 3 *and* daughter 4 *and* daughter 5)
= $0.5 \times 0.5 \times 0.5 \times 0.5 \times 0.5 = 0.03125$

However, the gender of the *next* baby is also an independent event, so, (surprisingly to some people!):

p (sixth child is a daughter) = 0.5

If we know the overall probabilities that anyone in our area is a wheelchair user or is a vegetarian, what is the probability that the next person to visit the clinic is both a wheelchair user and a vegetarian? We can assume that wheelchair use and vegetarianism are independent events. Thus if we know the probability that a person from among the clinic's clientele uses a wheelchair, and the probability that someone who uses the clinic is a vegetarian, we can *multiply* the figures together to find the probability that 'the next person to visit the clinic is a vegetarian wheelchair-user'.

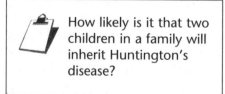

What is the chance of a vegetarian wheelchair user?

Suppose we want the probability that a female patient is potentially capable of child-bearing: how can we calculate the probability that a woman is either pregnant or infertile? The events 'the woman is pregnant' and 'the woman is infertile' cannot occur in the same person so they are mutually exclusive. Thus to find the probability of the combined event 'the woman is either pregnant or she is infertile' we *add* the individual probabilities. Taking this a stage further, the event 'the woman is pregnant, or infertile, or capable of child-bearing' is a 'dead cert' and so has probability 'one'.

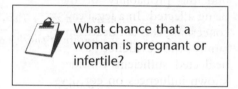

What chance that a woman is pregnant or infertile?

If we know the probability of a hereditary condition affecting one child in a family, what is the probability that a second or third child is affected? This matter of finding the probability of a second or third child in a family inheriting a particular condition is one that we must deal with very carefully indeed.

The transmission of genetic conditions from parent to child can vary according to different circumstances, but it is generally accepted that the probability of a child inheriting Huntington's disease from an afflicted parent is about 0.5. For this condition it is known that the health of each child is an independent event; so one child may inherit Huntington's disease but this is quite independent of whether or not their siblings also inherit the disease.

How likely is it that two children in a family will inherit Huntington's disease?

Suppose we select two children from the population of children having a parent with Huntington's disease: whether one child suffers from the disease is independent of whether the other suffers from it, so the probability that they *both* suffer from it is obtained by multiplication:

p (*both* children suffer from Huntington's disease) = 0.5 × 0.5 = 0.25

Similarly, if we know that the probability of anyone in the general population having Huntington's disease is 'h', say, and we pick two people at random, then:

p (*both* people suffer from Huntington's disease) = h × h = h²

However, we cannot assume that all health-related conditions occur as independent events: when one child in a family already has a certain condition there is a chance that the whole family is susceptible to that condition (whether due to heredity, environment or some other factor). In the absence of evidence to the contrary, we must allow the possibility that a second child having the same condition is *not* an independent event, and we must *not* use multiplication to find the probability of them both being affected. In a legal case in 1999 concerning two cot deaths in the same family the evidence as presented neglected sufficient consideration of known influences on cot deaths such

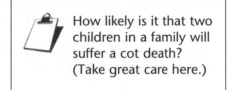

How likely is it that two children in a family will suffer a cot death? (Take great care here.)

as genetics, sleeping positions, heavy bedding and social circumstances. A major error was made by assuming that two cot deaths would be essentially independent events and, partly as a result, a mother was unjustly convicted of murder and imprisoned.

We cannot deduce a specific reaction from a general probability.

In the final question, if the overall probability of an allergic reaction to a particular drug is known, what is the probability of a woman being allergic? or a teenager? or a baby? If all we know is the *overall probability* of an allergic reaction to a particular drug then it is impossible, without further research, to calculate the *specific probabilities* of an allergic reaction which might be suffered by different subsets of people. More work is necessary.

7.3 Probabilities from z-scores

Now that we have some understanding of probability, and a feeling for what it means, we use these ideas in the context of the normal distributions of Sections 6.3 and 6.4. Our aim is to be able to determine when a value 'probably' does (or does not) belong to the given distribution, as this will allow us to conclude that 'probably' an assumption we have made is justified (or unjustified).

When dealing with the normal distribution we know that its curve is an example of a (smoothed off) histogram and the *area* under such a curve denotes frequency (see Figure 6.2). Up until now the vertical axis measures *frequency density*, but for this more generalised work we identify 'relative frequency' with 'probability', so from now on we let the vertical axis denote **probability density, p.d.** As already mentioned, once we have *standardised* a normal distribution then the total area under the curve is 'one': this fact allows us to calculate proportions easily as we did in Section 6.4. From now on we deal with the standardised normal curve $N(0,1^2)$ shown in Figure 7.1(a). It has mean $\mu = 0$, standard deviation $\sigma = 1$, and the total area under the curve is 'one', which is the total probability of 'all possible outcomes' and matches up with the idea that the probability of a 'dead cert' is 'one'. We interpret each section of area under the curve as a probability, so we can now use the table of the standard normal distribution (Appendix 5(b)) to give us these probabilities. In Figure 7.1(b) the *probability* of 'z' taking a value less than '0.8' is '1 – 0.2119', that is '0.7881':

p(z < 0.8) = 0.7881

The *probability* that 'z' lies between '–1' and '1.5' is '1 – 0.0668 – 0.1587', that is '0.7745' (Figure 7.1(c)):

p(–1 < z < 1.5) = 0.7745

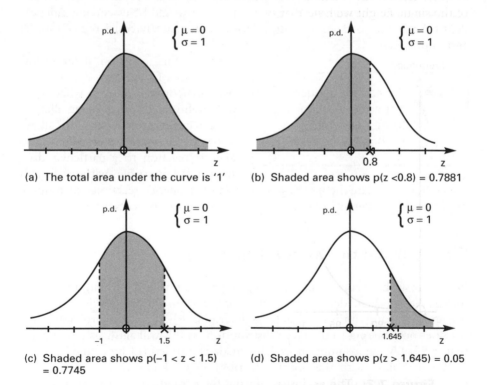

(a) The total area under the curve is '1'

(b) Shaded area shows p(z <0.8) = 0.7881

(c) Shaded area shows p(–1 < z < 1.5) = 0.7745

(d) Shaded area shows p(z > 1.645) = 0.05

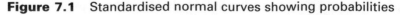

Figure 7.1   Standardised normal curves showing probabilities

The *probability* that 'z' is greater than '1.645' is '0.05' (Figure 7.1(d)):

$$p(z > 1.645) = 0.05$$

7.4 Hypothesis testing

We are now in a position to test if an assumption is 'probably justified'. Suppose we start with the assumption that 'the heights of all four-year-old boys in the UK form a normally distributed population with a mean value of $\mu = 102.4$ cm and a standard deviation of $\sigma = 4$ cm' (see Figure 7.2). We wish to *test* this assumption – is it *probably* justified? Since we cannot measure the heights of

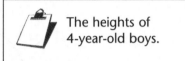

The heights of 4-year-old boys.

all four-year-old boys (quite impractical!), we measure the height of *one* four-year-old boy, *chosen at random*, and use that single value to test the validity of the assumption.

We begin by standardising this normal distribution of heights (Figure 7.3(a)). Then by the method of Section 6.4 we calculate the z-score (call it z_0) of the single height we have been able to measure: z_0 will fit somewhere along

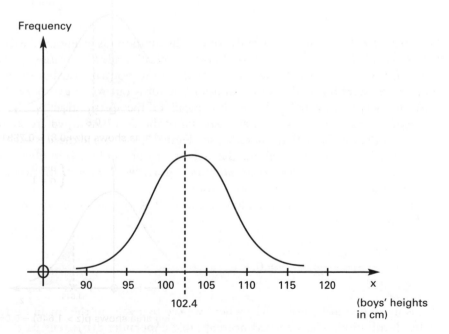

Figure 7.2 The assumed normal distribution of four-year-old boys' heights

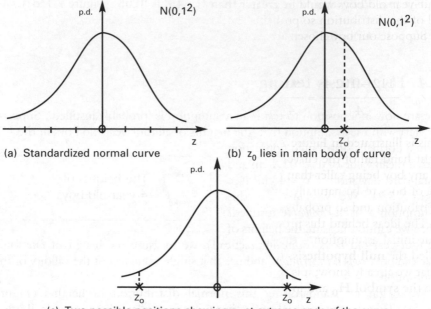

Figures 7.3 Possible positions of z_0 on the standardised normal curve

the z-axis. If z_0 lies in the 'main body' of the distribution (as in Figure 7.3(b)) then, since it is *likely* that our 'random' boy is 'typical', *probably our assumption is justified*; we are probably dealing with the same normal distribution we thought we were. But perhaps our random boy turns out to be exceptionally short or exceptionally tall – he is 'untypical' of the distribution we have assumed. In this case z_0 lies at an *extreme end* of the distribution, where there is a *very small* probability that values lie, see Figure 7.3(c). Since there is such a low probability of this happening, the height of our random boy does *not* support our basic assumption so *probably our assumption is unjustified*; we are probably dealing with a different distribution.

Suppose our boy chosen at random is exactly 104 cm tall. The z-score for this height is:

$$z_0 = \frac{104 - 102.4}{4} = \frac{1.6}{4} = 0.4$$

This is illustrated in Figure 7.3(b) where we see that z_0 is in the 'main body' of the distribution. The standard normal table (Appendix 5(b)) tells us that, on our assumption, there is a probability of 0.3446 of any boy being taller than this value; in other words we would naturally expect that more than a third of four-year-old boys would be taller than this anyway – the boy seems quite typical of the distribution so probably our assumption is justified.

Suppose our boy chosen at random is 112 cm tall. The z-score for this height is:

$$z_0 = \frac{112 - 102.4}{4} = \frac{9.6}{4} = 2.4$$

This is illustrated in Figure 7.3(c), where the position of z_0 is tucked under the right-hand tail of the curve. From Appendix 5(b) we read that the probability of any boy being taller than this is only 0.0082, so we would expect fewer than 1% of boys to be naturally taller than this. The boy is *exceptionally* tall for our distribution and so probably our assumption is unjustified.

The ideas behind this process are used in many types of **hypothesis testing**. Our initial assumption – the one that we would usually 'like' to be valid – is called the **null hypothesis**. It is called this because it implies 'no change' from what we already know; it is the 'status quo' position. For the null hypothesis we use the **symbol H_0** and in the above example we have:

'by H_0 the distribution of heights is $N(102.4, 4^2)$'

If the null hypothesis is not valid, then the **alternative hypothesis**, for which we use the **symbol H_1**, must be valid. H_1 does *not describe* any different distribution, it merely states that the null hypothesis is not valid. Thus in our example:

'by H_1 the distribution of heights is *not* $N(102.4, 4^2)$'

We do all calculations on the basis of the null hypothesis; it is only if we deduce that the null hypothesis is probably not valid that we 'accept' the alternative hypothesis.

From the outset of any hypothesis testing, we must decide precisely what we mean by 'extreme values' on our standardised graph. By convention, when the probability of an occurrence is *less than 5%*, that is, less than 0.05 or less than '1 in 20', then that event is extremely unlikely. Using this figure, we obtain results valid at the 5% **significance level**. (Other levels of significance exist, for example 10% which gives results at a weaker level of significance, or 1% which gives results at a stronger level of significance; 5% is the level most commonly used.) If extreme values might occur at *either end* of the distribution (our random boy could be exceptionally short *or* exceptionally tall) then the total probability of heights that are 'extra short' or 'extra tall' must add together to make 5% of the whole probability. Thus the areas symmetrically placed under the two 'tails' of the curve must together form 5% of the whole area (see Figure 7.4). These two areas combine to form the **critical region** under the curve (this

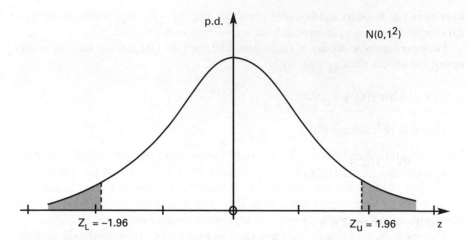

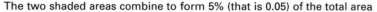

The two shaded areas combine to form 5% (that is 0.05) of the total area

Figure 7.4   The 5% critical region for a two-tailed test,
showing z_L and z_U

arrangement implies a **two-tailed test**, see Section 9.6 for more discussion of this point). If any value lies in the critical region then it means that the probability of that value occurring is 5% or less.

When we apply a two-tailed test at the 5% level of significance, we mark the z-scores which are the limits of the critical region on the standardised graph. As shown in Figure 7.4, 'z_L' is the limit of the left-hand tail and 'z_U' is the limit of the right-hand tail; the probability that any value in the distribution is less than z_L is 2½%, and the probability that any value in the distribution is more than z_U is also 2½%. From Appendix 5(b) we see that at the 5% level, $z_L = -1.96$ and $z_U = 1.96$. Thus the total probability of the occurrence of any value that is less than -1.96 or more than 1.96 is 5% or less.

Returning to the height of our randomly selected boy: if the boy's height is 105 cm, then (as in Section 6.4) we calculate:

$$z_0 = \frac{105 - 102.4}{4} = 0.65$$

Since:

$$-1.96 < 0.65 < 1.96$$

we have $z_L < z_0 < z_U$

and so the value of z_0 lies between z_L and z_U in the 'main body' of the distribution. Thus on the basis of this evidence we can conclude that our null hypothesis is *probably* valid, and, at the 5% significance level, we *accept the null hypothesis.*

However, maybe we have a situation where z_0 lies in the critical region by being either less than z_L or greater than z_U, that is:

$$z_0 < z_L \quad \text{or} \quad z_0 > z_U$$

This will be the case if the boy's height is 92cm, from which we calculate:

$$z_0 = \frac{92 - 102.4}{4} = -2.6$$

and we see that $-2.6 < -1.96$

In this case, at the 5% significance level we *reject the null hypothesis* and *accept the alternative hypothesis*: we deduce that the null hypothesis is *probably not* valid.

When we test the validity of a hypothesis like this the level of significance used is a crucial feature. The significance level corresponds to the level of probability at which the null hypothesis is rejected in favour of the alternative hypothesis, thus these techniques are often called **significance tests**.

In Chapter 9 we include some more specific examples on significance testing, and also discuss (see Section 9.6) occasions when a **one-tailed test** can be appropriate.

7.5 Possible errors

Significance testing is based on probabilities, so it cannot give results that are guaranteed accurate on every specific occasion.

Returning to the example introduced in the last Section when we chose the four-year-old boy at random: if he turned out to be exceptionally tall (say) and the z-score of his height did lie in the critical region, maybe – even so – our assumed normal population of heights *was the correct one*. It is possible that his height *did* belong to the assumed population, but by chance it was an extreme 'outlier' (some boy, some-where, is the tallest four-year-old of all!). In this case, our calculation

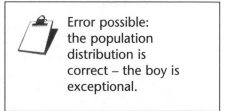

Error possible: the population distribution is correct – the boy is exceptional.

would have led us to reject the null hypothesis even though it was valid. We cannot avoid the fact that if an extreme value comes up, as a fluke, we might be led to reject the null hypothesis even when it is valid: this is called a **type I**

error. We must be aware of the possibility of type I errors but we cannot guarantee to avoid them; *the probability of a type I error is the same as the significance level* (thus, in the above examples there is a 5% probability of a type I error). The **symbol** α (written 'alpha', the Greek letter 'a') is often used to indicate the level of significance and also the probability of a type I error.

An undetected type I error could have serious consequences in clinical practice. The fluke recovery of a few patients might cause us to believe that an innovative treatment is effective, when in fact it is not; this could result in resources being wasted on worthless treatments.

> A clinical judgement for change, based on exceptional cases, might lead to wastage – or worse.

A **type II** error occurs if we accept a null hypothesis when it is not valid and we should be rejecting it. In our example the height of the randomly chosen boy might have fallen squarely in the 'main body' of our assumed distribution – and yet, in fact, this might have been an accidental occurrence, with the true distribution of heights being quite different. The probability of a type II error cannot be calculated unless we identify an alternative hypothesis more specifically; it is not a trivial matter to deal with this.

> Error possible: despite our example, the population distribution is different.

The **symbol** β (written 'beta', the Greek letter 'b') is sometimes used for the probability of a type II error, the probability that we accept a false null hypothesis. '$1 - \beta$' is thus the probability that we *reject* a false null hypothesis, that is we make a correct decision; '$1 - \beta$' is called the **power** of the significance test.

The clinical implication of a type II error might be that an ineffectual remedy continues to be applied, in the mistaken belief that it is more effective than a new development.

> This error might lead to a clinical judgement not to change to a superior treatment.

Estimating with Confidence

– using sample data to estimate the mean of a population

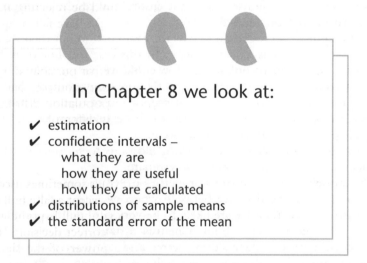

In Chapter 8 we look at:

✔ estimation
✔ confidence intervals –
    what they are
    how they are useful
    how they are calculated
✔ distributions of sample means
✔ the standard error of the mean

In all walks of life **estimation** is an essential skill. Among other things we need estimates of how long our journey to work will take, what quantity of sterile equipment to order from stores each month and what is the likely number of patients that can be seen in an Out-patients Department in a day. While we use descriptive statistics in gathering data and in sorting, displaying and summarising data (often resulting in very precise numbers), the *purpose* of using statistical tools is often to supply the evidence on which we can confidently base estimates.

In practical work and in research we usually seek to make *overall* descriptions, to compare distributions *in general terms*, and to *estimate* the likelihood of a particular outcome. Even when every measurement is reliable and our calculations are accurate, our purpose is all about **estimating**, essentially guessing or approximating. Our calculations result in figures which allow us to compare one guess with another, or to say how good a guess is likely to be – this is called **inferential statistics**.

We use the figures to quantify our **confidence** that an estimate is a good one, or that a guess is likely to be valid. For example, using data from a sample we can state the probability that the mean of the population from which the sample is drawn lies within a particular estimated range.

8.1 Confidence

We all have an idea of what is meant by **confidence**. If we work hard for an examination then we may be reasonably confident that we will pass it; if we practice hard at a sport then we may be confident that we will succeed in it. However 'confidence' by itself does not ensure any result: unfortunately we may fail that examination and lose that race!

If we thought we were certain to pass the examination but then we failed it, we could be described as 'overconfident'. In this case we should try to judge the basis for our assumed confidence. How could we have measured our confidence? We could have asked ourselves exactly how many hours we had studied, what was the quality of our study, what proportion of topics we had covered, what was the usual pass rate – answers to those questions would give us a measurement of just how confident we were.

In Statistics, the concept of confidence allows us to *measure* just how sure (confident) we are in a prediction or an estimate.

There are several fairly obvious properties of 'confidence'. For example, if we try to estimate the distance between where we are standing and a wall several metres away, then we are likely to be very confident in estimating the distance in whole metres: 'about 5 metres distant'. However, it is much harder to estimate this distance in metres and centimetres, to the nearest centimetre, and as a result we will be much less confident in our answer. The point is that the more accurate we try to be, the less confident we are in our estimate. Returning to our examination: we may be fairly confident that we will pass it, but much less confident about the exact mark we will obtain.

 Estimating how many men on a mixed sex ward.

Another property of 'confidence' is illustrated by the following example. We imagine that we are trying to estimate the number of men on a mixed-sex, 30 bed, surgical ward. The least possible number is 'zero' and the largest possible number is '30'. By ascertaining the sex of the patient in each bed we begin to refine these limits. If the patient in the first bed is male then our estimate for the total number of men narrows slightly to 'between 1 and 30'; if the patient in the second bed is female

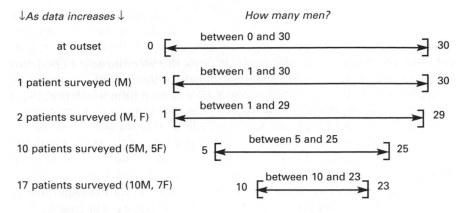

Figure 8.1 More data gives more accuracy in an estimate

then our estimate becomes 'between 1 and 29'. If we identify the first ten patients to be five men and five women, then we know that the total number of men lies 'between 5 and 25'; if the first seventeen patients are ten men and seven women, then we estimate the total number of men to be 'between 10 and 23'. The more patients whose sex we are sure of, the closer our estimate gets to the actual total of men on the ward. In the end, when we have found the sex of every patient, then we know precisely how many men there are – and we are completely confident in that number. As indicated in Figure 8.1, our confidence in our estimate grows as we gain more data. This is generally true – the more data we use in making an estimate, then the more confidence we have in that estimate.

When dealing with the sequence of estimates in the above example, we expressed each estimate as a **confidence interval**: 'we believe the number lies between 10 and 23', etc. But the wider the confidence interval was, the less precise we could be about the *actual* value we were seeking. In this simple example the estimates were obviously unnecessary: in the end we could find the precise number of men in the ward just by counting. However, in many situations we are unable to 'just count' the number we require; in these cases estimation is essential and the use of confidence intervals is a crucial tool. In the following sections we illustrate this use, showing how we can obtain a confidence interval for the (otherwise inaccessible) mean of a population.

8.2 Unbiased estimators

Before we look at the levels of confidence we can have in approximations, we consider the basic, rough and ready figures that might occur to us. If we have access to data from a suitable sample then we can calculate the sample mean, $\bar{x}$, and we are generally entitled to take this value as a first approximation to μ, the population mean. So we have:

$$\mu \approx \bar{x}$$

where the symbol '$\approx$' means 'is approximately equal to'. We say that '$\bar{x}$' is an **unbiased estimator** for 'μ'. (However, because this value is likely to be rather inaccurate, we often prefer to obtain a confidence interval for μ.)

Approximating the population variance (σ^2) from a sample variance (s^2) is not quite so straightforward. Variance is a measure of dispersion or 'spread-out-ness' (see Section 5.3), and common sense tells us that the spread-out-ness of a sample is likely to *underestimate* the spread-out-ness of the population. This is because a random sample will probably not include all the extreme values in the population. To take account of this we increase the sample variance (s^2) by 'scaling it up' in order to obtain an approximation for the population variance. The scale factor that has been found to work best is:

$$\frac{n}{n-1}$$

based on the size 'n' of the sample (with the top of the fraction larger than the bottom, this number is necessarily greater than 'one' so it is bound to *increase* the value). So we say that σ^2 is approximately the same as:

$$\left(\frac{n}{n-1}\right) s^2, \text{ that is:}$$

$$\sigma^2 \approx \left(\frac{n}{n-1}\right) s^2$$

Thus '$\left(\dfrac{n}{n-1}\right) s^2$ ' is an *unbiased estimator* for σ^2

Because variance and standard deviation are so closely related, we can immediately write down an approximation for the population standard deviation, σ, using a sample standard deviation, s:

$$\sigma \approx \sqrt{\frac{n}{n-1}}\, s$$

and we say that:

'$\dfrac{n}{n-1}\, s$ ' is an *unbiased estimator* for σ^2

8.3 The distribution of sample means

In Section 6.3 we met the normal distribution of a population, $N(\mu, \sigma^2)$, characterised by its mean, μ, and its variance, σ^2. In practice it is unlikely that we ever use this distribution just as it is, since we rarely have access to a *whole population* of anything. Usually, as discussed in Chapter 3, we take *samples* from a population, and from measurements made on the samples we estimate the corresponding measurement for the population.

Suppose we wish to know the mean blood potassium level of all people taking potassium sparing diuretics – then we cannot possibly test the blood of *all* people taking diuretics, not even of all of those in one NHS Trust. Instead we can obtain a *sample* of people taking these potassium sparing diuretics, and find the mean blood

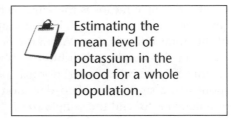 Estimating the mean level of potassium in the blood for a whole population.

potassium level for this sample of people. The question then is, *how close* is our sample mean likely to be to the population mean? Putting this another way, how *confident* can we be that our sample mean can be used as an estimate for the true mean of the population?

Of course, we could take a selection of different samples, each of 'n' individuals, from our population (assumed to be normally distributed). From each sample we could calculate the mean blood potassium level for the people concerned. We would find that these mean values themselves are normally distributed: the **distribution of the sample means** is normal (see Figure 8.2)

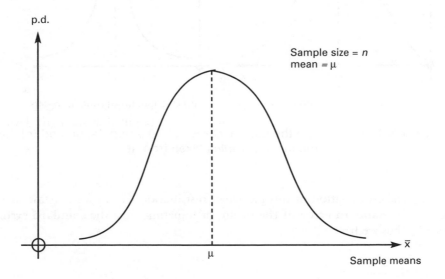

Figure 8.2   The distribution of sample means

and the mean of this distribution is *the same* as the population mean. But none of the samples we deal with is likely to give us exactly the same mean value for blood potassium levels as the population mean: some of our sample means will be higher than the population mean and some will be lower. The best we can hope for is to find an **interval estimate** for the population mean, that is a range of values within which the population mean 'probably' lies. So the question remains: using the mean from just one sample, can we find a confidence interval for the population mean? – can we find its **confidence limits**?

Using the notation of Section 5.2 we call a sample mean x̄; since the mean of all the sample means is the same as the population mean, in Figure 8.2 we label the overall mean as 'μ'. This **sampling distribution** has the overall shape of the normal distribution. When the population is also normal we see that the curve for the sampling distribution is 'narrower' than that for the population (Figure 8.3). This 'narrower' normal curve for the sampling distribution corresponds to a smaller standard deviation. When the standard deviation of the population is 'σ' and the sample size is 'n', the standard deviation of the distribution of sample means is given by:

$$\text{standard deviation of sample means} = \frac{\sigma}{\sqrt{n}}$$

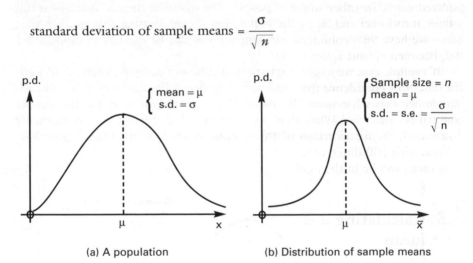

(a) A population   (b) Distribution of sample means

Figure 8.3   Comparing the normal curves of (a) a population and (b) the means of samples taken from it

This standard deviation of this particular distribution has a special name: it is called the **standard error of the mean**, or sometimes just the **standard error** (s.e.). Thus we have:

$$\text{s.e.} = \frac{\sigma}{\sqrt{n}}$$

We must not confuse the terms 'standard deviation' – which can be applied to *any* distribution – and 'standard error', which is only used for sampling distributions. It is by using this standard error that we can measure our confidence that a population mean is close to any particular sample mean: standard errors allow us to calculate confidence intervals.

8.4 Confidence intervals for population means

In this section we use a confidence interval to state 'how confident' we are that we can estimate the (unknown) mean of a population by using the mean of a single sample. Repeated sampling *could* be used, but that would be unusual – and costly! (Dealing with one sample is usually quite onerous enough!)

From a single sample (of size n) we calculate the sample mean, $\bar{x}$, and the sample standard deviation, s. From these we estimate the population standard deviation, σ, and hence the standard error, s.e. These allow us to calculate how confident we are that the population mean, μ, lies within a range of values centred on $\bar{x}$. In other words, we find a certain interval (by determining the values at its lower end, $\bar{x}_L$, and upper end, $\bar{x}_U$) and we can say that – for example – we have 95% confidence that the population mean lies within this interval, between $\bar{x}_L$ and $\bar{x}_U$.

In a simple case we might conclude that, while the mean of our sample is '9', we have 95% confidence that our population mean lies 'between 2 and 16'. We remember that what we are doing is *estimating* an interval within which the population mean lies. While there are no guarantees that the sample we happen to choose will give an accurate interval, we are confident that if we do this estimation with 100 different samples then in 95 out of the 100 cases the population mean will lie in the interval we obtain.

8.5 Calculating a confidence interval for a population mean

As mentioned above in Section 8.3, when a population is known to be 'normal' then the distribution of sample means is also normal. In fact if the size of sample is large enough (generally taken to be 'more than 30') then *whatever* the underlying distribution is we can assume that the distribution of sample means is normal. Thus in most cases we use the methods of Chapter 7, concerning normal distributions, to calculate the interval estimate for a population mean.

We first take a sample of size n, and calculate the mean value for this sample, $\bar{x}$, and also its standard deviation, s (see Sections 5.2 and 5.3). While we have no hard information about the population as a whole, we use these figures to obtain an unbiased estimate for the standard deviation of the population, namely:

$$\sigma \approx s \sqrt{\frac{n}{n-1}} \text{ (see Section 8.2).}$$

Our purpose is to estimate an interval within which the population mean, μ, lies. We assume that the distribution of all the sample means is normal, with mean μ; the standard error is:

$$\text{s.e.} = \frac{\sigma}{\sqrt{n}} \text{ (see Section 8.3). In fact, since we have:}$$

$$\text{s.e.} = \frac{\sigma}{\sqrt{n}} = \frac{1}{\sqrt{n}} \times \sigma$$

we also have:

$$\text{s.e.} \approx \frac{1}{\sqrt{n}} \times s \sqrt{\frac{n}{n-1}} = \frac{s}{\sqrt{n-1}}$$

which means we can estimate the standard error from the sample standard deviation we have calculated. Table 8.1 summarises these facts.

Table 8.1   Summary of statistics and parameters

Sample	Population	Distribution of sample means
size = n, by design		
mean = $\bar{x}$, calculated	mean = μ, unknown	mean = μ, assumed
s.d. = s, calculated	s.d. = σ, unknown	s.e. = $\dfrac{\sigma}{\sqrt{n}}$, estimated
	& $\sigma = s \sqrt{\dfrac{n}{n-1}}$, estimated	s.e. = $\dfrac{s}{\sqrt{n-1}}$, estimated

Using the figures n, $\bar{x}$ and s that we suppose we know, we wish to calculate 95% confidence limits for the population mean μ by considering the (normal) distribution of the sample means, see Figure 8.4. We first need the values of the lower and upper limits, $\bar{x}_L$ and $\bar{x}_U$, such that 2½% of this distribution lies *below* $\bar{x}_L$, and 2½% of the distribution lies *above* $\bar{x}_U$; then the central interval between $\bar{x}_L$ and $\bar{x}_U$ includes 95% of the distribution.

When we deal with the *standardised* normal curve for the sample means (see Figure 8.5) then 95% of the area under this curve, symmetrically around the mean (= 0), is included between the z-scores shown. The values of z_L and z_U

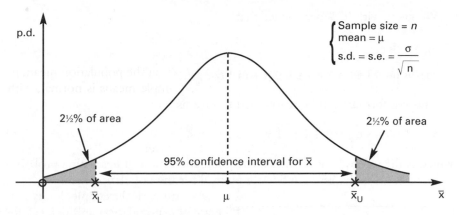

Figure 8.4 The normal distribution of sample means

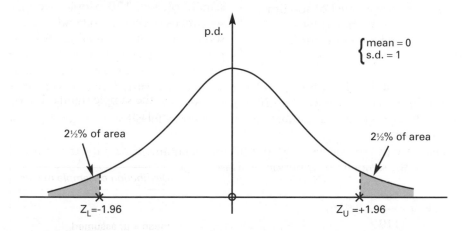

Figure 8.5 The standardised normal curve for sample means

are obtained from Appendix 5(b): z_L = –1.96 because the area below z_L is 0.025 (or 2½%) of the whole; z_U = 1.96 because the area above z_U is 0.025 (or 2½%) of the whole. We remember that the areas represent probabilities.

We now use these values of z_L and z_U to 'work backwards' to find the values of $\bar{x}_L$ and $\bar{x}_L$, using a formula that corresponds to that in Section 6.4:

$$z = \frac{\bar{x} - \mu}{s.e.}$$

Thus $-1.96 = \dfrac{\bar{x}_L - \mu}{s.e.}$ so $= \bar{x}_L = \mu - (1.96 \times s.e.)$

and similarly $\bar{x}_U = \mu + (1.96 \times s.e.)$

We know with 95% confidence that:

$$\bar{x}_L \leq \bar{x} \leq \bar{x}_U$$

that is $\mu - (1.96 \times \text{s.e.}) \leq \bar{x} \leq \mu + (1.96 \times \text{s.e.})$

This last formula can be rearranged to give us:

$$\bar{x} - (1.96 \times \text{s.e.}) \leq \mu \leq \bar{x} + (1.96 \times \text{s.e.}) \qquad (*)$$

which is the interval within which the population mean μ lies with a probability of 95% – it is the 95% confidence interval for the population mean.

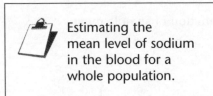

Estimating the mean level of sodium in the blood for a whole population.

As a numerical example, let us estimate the population mean level for blood sodium. Having chosen a sample of, say, 120 people, we take specimens of their blood and find the sodium content, in milli-equivalents per litre, of each specimen. For these 120 values we calculate the sample mean (say it is 140 mEq/l) and the sample standard deviation (say it is 10 mEq/l). Thus we have n = 120, $\bar{x}$ = 140 and s = 10; from these figures we can calculate an interval estimate for μ, the mean blood sodium level *for the population*.

First we use the values of 's' and 'n' to obtain an estimate for the standard error of the sampling distribution. This is:

$$\text{s.e.} = \frac{10}{\sqrt{119}} = 0.9167$$

We take s.e. = 0.92, correct to two decimal places.

If we want a 95% confidence limit for the population mean, then corresponding to the probability values of 0.025 (that is 2½%) under each 'tail' of the curve, Appendix 5(b) gives us the z-values of ±1.96. Using the (*) formula from above:

$$\bar{x} - (1.96 \times \text{s.e.}) \leq \mu \leq \bar{x} + (1.96 \times \text{s.e.})$$

so the 95% confidence limits in this case are:

$$140 - (1.96 \times 0.92) \leq \mu \leq 140 + (1.96 \times 0.92)$$

that is:

$$138.20 \leq \mu \leq 141.80$$

using 2 decimal places throughout.

Thus in estimating the mean blood sodium level for the population we know that there is a probability of 95% that this population mean lies between 138.20 mEq/l and 141.80 mEq/l.

Suppose we wish to refine this estimate, and obtain an interval which we can be 99% sure will contain the population mean?

> A more confident estimate for the population mean level for blood sodium.

In this case the proportion of area/probability under each 'tail' of the curve is 0.005 (that is 0.5%), so Appendix 5(b) gives us $z_L = -2.58$ and $z_U = +2.58$. We use the same (*) formula, which gives:

$$\bar{x} - (2.58 \times \text{s.e.}) \leq \mu \leq \bar{x} + (2.58 \times \text{s.e.})$$

Putting in our values for and s.e. we have:

$$140 - (2.58 \times 0.92) \leq \mu \leq 140 + (2.58 \times 0.92)$$

so that:

$$137.63 \leq \mu \leq 142.37$$

The interval estimate for the population mean of blood sodium content (with 99% confidence) is thus between 137.63 mEq/l and 142.37 mEq/l.

Since, in this second case we want to be *more* confident that the interval contains the population mean, the interval we obtain is wider – we have *less* accuracy. This is generally true, and corresponds with the 'distance from a wall' example in Section 8.1: the *higher* the required level of confidence in our estimate, the *lower* the precision of that estimate. There is always a trade-off to be made between our desired level of confidence and the appropriate degree of accuracy in our estimate.

Normal or Not?

– *using z-scores and t-scores to test if samples come from known populations*

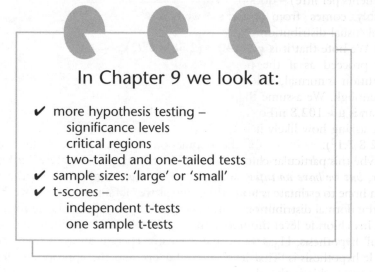

In Chapter 9 we look at:

✔ more hypothesis testing –
significance levels
critical regions
two-tailed and one-tailed tests
✔ sample sizes: 'large' or 'small'
✔ t-scores –
independent t-tests
one sample t-tests

In many clinical situations we may wish to test a hypothesis, for example 'Patients given drug X do better than those given the accepted 'best available' drug'. In many cases it is also important that we can *quantify* the likelihood that this hypothesis is valid. So now we look at practical aspects of **hypothesis testing**, where inferential statistics gives us tools to estimate whether samples come from a known (normal) distribution, or some other. As we show, we can test the validity of hypotheses *and* we can quantify the level of certainty to be given to our results.

In the previous chapter we used information about the mean of a sample to estimate the mean of the population *from which the sample came*. We now look at these matters from a slightly different point of view: how can we decide the probability that any particular value, or given sample, is really likely to have come from a specific population?

9.1 A sample-of-one: is it normal?

As in the example in Section 7.4, it is often useful to estimate whether a single value or reading, a **sample-of-one**, really does come from the 'population' that we know about. In other words, is this value probably part of the *known population* (so we can safely make deductions about it) or is it (probably) part of a quite different distribution?

To illustrate this with a clinical example we ask whether we should consider the level of chloride in serum taken from a newborn child to be **abnormal** if the reading is 112 mEq/l (milli-Equivalents per litre) – does this value probably comes from *outside* the normal/usual distribution of chloride levels? We note that it is *quite safe* for us to proceed as if the population distribution *is* normal, as long as it is large enough. We assume that we have information about the population: say its mean is μ = 102.8 mEq/l and its standard deviation is σ = 7.1 mEq/l. Thus we are asking how likely it is that a value of '112' belongs to the distribution $N(102.8, 7.1^2)$.

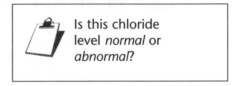

Is this chloride level *normal* or *abnormal*?

Maybe this particular chloride level comes from a different distribution altogether, *but we have no information at all about any other such distribution.* All we can hope to estimate is how probable it is that the given chloride level comes from the normal distribution we know about. So our task is to test the hypothesis 'This chloride level *does* come from the given normal distribution'; this is the null hypothesis, H_0: *'there is no change; things are as we expect'*. The other possible hypothesis is 'This chloride level does *not* come from the given normal distribution'; this is the alternative hypothesis, H_1: *'things are different from expected'*. The conclusion we get depends on the significance level that we require in the answer; suppose we wish to test that '112' comes from the distribution, $N(102.8, 7.1^2)$ and we want the result to be *significant at the 5% level* (say).

The null hypothesis is that x = 112 comes from $N(102.8, 7.1^2)$, so we calculate the z-score for this value (see Section 6.4):

$$z = \frac{x - \mu}{\sigma} = \frac{112 - 102.8}{7.1} = \frac{9.2}{7.1} = 1.3$$

This score is shown on the standard normal curve in Figure 9.1.

Now we wish to be able to state at the 5% significance level whether '112'

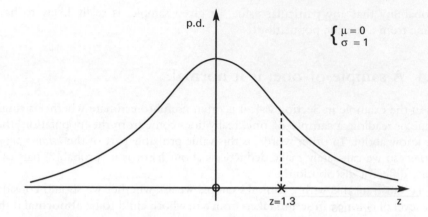

Figure 9.1   The z-score for the single sample of serum

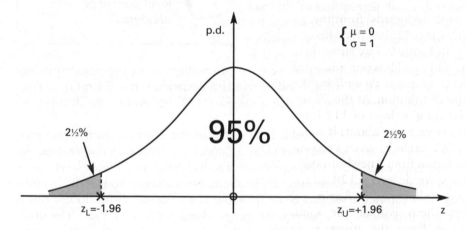

Figure 9.2   The critical region at 5% significance on a standard normal curve (two-tailed test)

belongs to $N(102.8, 7.1^2)$. This means that we will *accept* the null hypothesis, that '112' belongs to this normal distribution, so long as '112' does *not* lie in the critical region of the graph. In this instance the 5% critical region gives the set of values which lie *outside* the 95% of the distribution centred on the mean.

In Figure 9.2, the 5% critical region is shown shaded (the two 'tails') and the rest of the area under the standard normal curve represents the 'central 95%' of the distribution; the z-scores z_L and z_U mark the limits of this area. Since the critical region is in two sections, our test score might be 'unacceptable' by being *either* too big (greater than z_U) *or* too small (less than z_L), thus this is a two-tailed test. Using the same method as in Sections 7.4 and 8.5 we

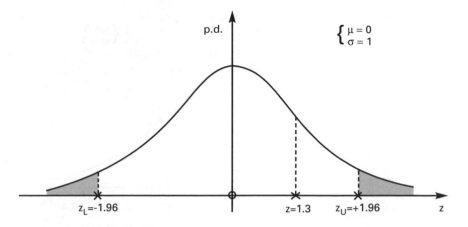

Figure 9.3   We accept the null hypothesis at 5% significance level

'work backwards' from the Table in Appendix 5(b). The area above z_U is 2½% (that is 0.025) of the whole. Thus $z_U = 1.96$ and by symmetry $z_L = -1.96$.

In Figure 9.3 we show the three z-scores and we see that $z = 1.3$ lies between z_L and z_U. Thus our z-score is *not* in the critical region, so at a 5% significance level *we accept the null hypothesis*: we say that $z = 1.3$ probably *does* belong to this distribution. At the 5% significance level we believe that our sample-of-one, the chloride level of 112 mEq/l, probably *does* come from the normal distribution we know about; it is *not* abnormal.

We might be given a second sample of serum from a newborn child, where the chloride level is 120 mEq/l: is this one 'abnormal'? Again our null hypothesis is that the sample *does* come from the given population, $N(102.8, 7.1^2)$, and we again work at

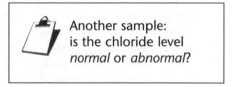

Another sample: is the chloride level *normal* or *abnormal?*

the 5% significance level (although significance levels of 1% and 0.1% would also be possible). We calculate the z-score corresponding to $x = 120$:

$$z = \frac{120 - 102.8}{7.1} = \frac{17.2}{7.1} = 2.4$$

In Figure 9.4 we show the diagram of the standard normal curve with the critical region indicated. Clearly the z-score '$z = 2.4$' falls within the critical region. This causes us to *reject* the null hypothesis, and *accept* the alternative hypothesis. We can*not* say (at the 5% significance level) that this sample comes from our known population. We identify the chloride level in the sample as 'probably abnormal', but we *cannot* say from which other distribution it might come.

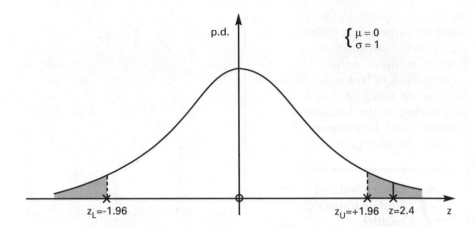

Figure 9.4   We reject the null hypothesis at 5% significance level

If we test a hypothesis in this way and find that a particular reading is 'abnormal', what clinical consequences might there be? The significance level we used here was '5%', so 'failing' this significance test means the likelihood that the reading is from the known normal population is less than 5 in 100, that is less than 1 in 20. But is this enough to persuade us that the reading *necessarily* comes from a different population and that some treatment might be needed? If we are not convinced, then we could make the conditions more demanding, by repeating the significance test at the '1%' level (or smaller). By itself, the fact that the level of chloride in the sample of serum is 'abnormal' in this sense (at 5% significance) does not give us enough information to be *certain* of the situation. This is why the idea of what is normal/usual in a clinical sense is often decided with a degree of arbitrariness, and described as a fairly wide range of possibilities. But if we regard a *very* wide range of possibilities as being normal/usual, then perhaps some patients with a really abnormal reading might go untreated! In most cases, clinical judgement of all the symptoms is still essential.

> How might a clinician react to an 'abnormal' result?

9.2 Differences between groups of people

Differences between groups of people, or between a group and the whole population, are usually judged *on differences between the means* of the conditions being measured, as we discuss in the following examples.

It is often useful to test for differences between a sample group of people and the whole population. An example is when we suspect that children growing up in the environment of nuclear power stations might have an increased risk of leukaemia: the mean number of cases of leukaemia per year arising in the locality of power

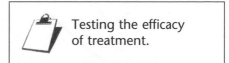

Can children be affected by growing up near a nuclear power station?

stations could be compared with the mean number per year in the whole country. Another example is to test whether the heights of a group of people living in an isolated community are significantly different from the heights of people in the adjacent town (this could be relevant for understanding their situation – malnutrition? inbreeding?). The analysis is done on the mean heights.

Can an isolated lifestyle impact on health?

A further example is in a clinical situation when we wish to test the efficacy of a particular treatment given to a sample group of people; the testing involves the means of measurements on both the sample and the population. In all these cases, whatever measurements are made, we compare the *mean of the sample* with the *mean of the population*.

Testing the efficacy of treatment.

Testing for a 'placebo effect' used to be one of the most common uses of statistics in medical trials, where it was used to compare two sample groups of patients. When a new medicine was being tested, such a trial was used to decide whether one group of patients was significantly improved compared with the other. The first group received the new drug, while the second group (the 'control group') received either no drug at all or a **placebo**, an inactive 'dummy drug'. For both groups the individu-

Placebos.

als' improvements were measured, then the difference between the groups was determined – *usually by comparing the mean values of the two samples*. Nowadays a placebo is rarely used in clinical trials – for ethical reasons. It is more common to compare two groups of patients where one group receives the new drug while the other receives the accepted 'best available' drug.

There are many other occasions when treatments and therapies used by nursing and other health professionals are evaluated by comparing two groups of people for significant differences. For example, tests for general health, or for response to a particular therapy, can be made on a group of men and a group of women, or a group of teenagers and a group of retired people. The treatments are evaluated by *comparing the mean values* of the relevant measurements from each sample group.

When we have taken measurements on sample groups of people such as those described above, our task is to compare *either* the mean of a sample with the mean of the population *or* the means of two different samples; however it is rarely sufficient just to look at the sizes of the two means involved. The mean of one group may be bigger than the mean of the other, but there may be *many* individuals in the second group whose individual measurements are bigger than the mean of the first group. It can appear to be quite difficult to disentangle the required result (see Figure 9.5).

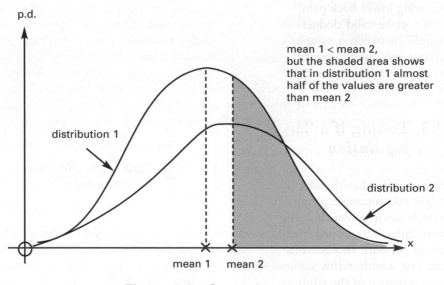

Figure 9.5   Comparing means

As a specific example, suppose we are investigating the efficacy of spinal manipulation for alleviating lower back pain. We can take two groups of people with lower back pain, apply spinal manipulation to one group but not to the other, then afterwards measure the levels of lower back pain in the individuals of both groups. We commonly measure 'Pain' using a scale with apparently equal intervals marked on it (as in Section 2.3, question 6); the patient rings a number on the scale to indicate the subjective level of pain they are experiencing. The mean score for the pain experienced by each group is calculated from each set of scores (see Section 5.2). If the mean score for pain is lower in the group who have had the spinal

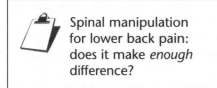

Spinal manipulation for lower back pain: does it make *enough* difference?

manipulation than in the other (control) group, then we may – or may not? – be justified in concluding that the spinal manipulation is effective.

The issue is in the nature of 'the mean'. Means are used to summarise data and it is rather unlikely that any individual in either group scores *exactly* the mean value: there will be individual values lying both above and below each mean. But the problem is that this is true of *both* groups. It is likely that there are individual scores from the control group which are less than some individual scores from those who have received treatment. And probably there are individuals who have had spinal manipulation who still score their pain higher than some individuals in the control group. How do we decide if the means are *different enough* for us to conclude that spinal manipulation is effective in reducing lower back pain?

To make valid deductions about significant differences between groups of people (between a sample and the population, or between two samples) we cannot rely merely on comparing the mean values; we *must* use appropriate hypothesis testing, as we show below.

9.3 Testing if a 'large' sample comes from a *known population*

In testing for health risks associated with a particular sedentary style of life we might take a sample group of 50 men, aged between 35 and 39, who all work long hours in a very desk-bound environment. We record the diastolic blood pressure of each man, and we can test whether this sample is truly representative of the adult male population as a whole. For adult men in this age group we take the population

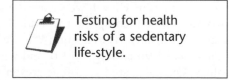

Testing for health risks of a sedentary life-style.

mean for diastolic blood pressure to be 80 mmHg and, similar to the situation in Section 9.1, we want to test the null hypothesis that 'this sample of blood pressures really does come from our known (normal) population distribution'. The alternative is that the sample is abnormal and comes from some other distribution, in which case there is the possibility that some interventions may be needed to maintain the men's health.

The sample size of '50' is carefully chosen. Any sample whose size is greater than '30', which comes from a fairly symmetrical population distribution, is generally called a **large sample**. (If the population distribution is very skewed, then we need a sample size of up to 200 before it is called 'large'.)

Using measurements from our sample group we calculate the mean for the sample, which we take to be 84 mmHg. Thus we have the sample mean $\bar{x} = 84$, which we wish to compare with the known mean of the population, $\mu = 80$, at a significance level of 5% (say). Now there are two possibilities to be considered:

we may or we may not know the precise value of the standard deviation of the population.

If we *do* know the population standard deviation (say σ = 10.4) then the calculation to test our null hypothesis is straightforward. We deal with the number $\bar{x}$ = 84 as a sample-of-one (as in Section 9.1) where the distribution is now the 'distribution of sample means', see Section 8.3. We know that the mean of this distribution of sample means is μ = 80 (like the underlying population). Since the standard error is:

$$\frac{\sigma}{\sqrt{n}}$$, where 'n = 50' is the size of the sample, we here have:

$$\text{s.e.} = \frac{10.4}{\sqrt{50}} = 1.47$$

We calculate the z-score for $\bar{x}$ = 84:

$$z = \frac{\bar{x} - \mu}{s.e.} = \frac{84 - 80}{1.47}$$

that is z = 2.72

(which is not difficult when we use a calculator). To test the null hypothesis at the 5% significance level, we sketch the standardised normal curve showing the two tails which comprise the critical region of 5% of the total area (see Figure 9.2 again). As in Section 9.1, we read from the Table in Appendix 5(b) that z_L = $-$ 1.96 and z_U = 1.96, and we compare the above z-score with these values. Our calculated z-score is greater than z_U:

$$2.72 \geq 1.96$$

so it lies in the critical region and we deduce that, at the 5% significance level, it is likely that our sample mean comes from 'some other' distribution of sample means. (If our z-score were *not* in the critical region then we would *accept* the null hypothesis and conclude that our sample of blood pressures probably *does* come from the known population we started with.)

If we do *not* know the population standard deviation, then the calculation to test our null hypothesis needs a small modification. We again deal with the number $\bar{x}$ = 84 as a sample-of-one from the distribution of sample means. As above, the mean of this distribution is μ = 80 (the underlying population mean). Since we do not know σ, we must estimate the standard error (see Section 8.3) from the sample standard deviation, s. If we calculate s to be 10 (say) and n = 50 we use the information in Table 8.1 to estimate:

$$\text{s.e.} = \frac{s}{\sqrt{n-1}} = \frac{10}{\sqrt{49}} = 1.43$$

Using this alternative estimate for the standard error, we calculate the z-score for $\bar{x} = 84$:

$$z = \frac{\bar{x} - \mu}{s.e.} = \frac{84 - 80}{1.43}$$

that is $z = 2.80$

We now test the null hypothesis at the 5% significance level. Since the calculated z-score is greater than $z_U = 1.96$ it is in the critical region. Thus, as in the above case, we deduce that this sample of blood pressures probably comes from a 'different distribution'.

In both of the above cases our calculations yield results which are significant at the 5% level. We deduce that this sample of men appears to be atypical of the population as a whole: their sedentary lifestyle may be a factor that needs addressing.

9.4 Testing if 'large' samples come from the *same population*

At first sight, this test appears similar to that described in Section 9.3. We imagine that we have two large groups of people (35 men and 45 women) and we wish to know whether their haemoglobin levels come from the same overall (normal) population. However, here we are assuming that we have no independent information about the mean of any underlying population of haemoglobin levels – we are testing merely whether the samples come from the *same population* (in a statistical

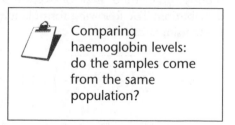

Comparing haemoglobin levels: do the samples come from the same population?

sense). If we happen to know the standard deviation of the population, then our test involves calculating a z-score, as before. If, as is rather more common, we do *not* know the standard deviation of the population, then we estimate it from the standard deviations of both samples, and apply a test using a **t-score**: this process is called an **independent t-test**.

We start by recording the haemoglobin levels in the two samples, in g/dl, and calculating the means and standard deviations of these levels for each sample. Suppose we have for the sample of men:

sample size = 35
mean = $\overline{x}_M$ = 14
standard deviation = s_M = 1.2

and for the sample of women:

sample size = 45
mean = $\overline{x}_w$ = 11
standard deviation = s_W = 1.0

We must allow for the possibility that these samples of haemoglobin levels come from different populations (statistically speaking): the first with mean μ_M and standard deviation σ_M, say, and the second with mean μ_W and standard deviation μ_W. However, we take as our null hypothesis that both samples actually do come from the same population, so the null hypothesis tells us that:

$\mu_M = \mu_W$, which we write as μ

and:

$\sigma_M = \sigma_W$, which write as σ (for simplicity)

The sample-of-one that we consider in this case is the value '$\overline{x}_M - \overline{x}_W$'. We test whether this gives a score that lies in the critical region under the curve, according to our pre-agreed level of significance (this part is similar to Section 9.3).

If we happen to know the value of 'σ', the standard deviation of the population, we continue as follows. Say we know that σ = 1.14, then we slightly modify the method used for Section 9.3 to obtain the standard error for our distribution. The following formula may look daunting but we can deal with it easily using a calculator:

$$\text{s.e.} = \sigma \sqrt{\left(\frac{1}{35} + \frac{1}{45}\right)} = 1.14 \times \sqrt{\left(\frac{1}{35} + \frac{1}{45}\right)}$$

Thus we obtain the standard error correct to 2 decimal places:

s.e. = 0.26

Using this value for the standard error, the z-score is:

$$z = \frac{(\overline{x}_M - \overline{x}_W) - (\mu - \mu)}{s.e.} = \frac{(14 - 11) - 0}{0.26} = 11.5$$

We 'work backwards' from the Table (Appendix 5(b)). At the 5% level of significance, the boundary of the 5% critical region is given by $z_u = 1.64$ (we have arranged that z must be positive, so only the right-hand tail is relevant). Obviously our calculated value is far greater than '1.64', so it is in the critical region. Thus we reject the null hypothesis: at the 5% significance level it is *unlikely* that the two samples come from the same population of haemoglobin levels.

If, as is more usual, we do not know the value of 'σ', we first obtain an estimate for σ before we can calculate the standard error. Our null hypothesis is that we are dealing with *only one population*. Thus we can find an estimate for σ by mentally 'pooling' the two samples into one larger sample (in fact the following method can be used for both 'large' and 'small' samples). Pooling the samples allows us to calculate an estimate for σ as:

$$\sigma = \sqrt{\frac{35s_M^2 + 45s_W^2}{35 + 45 - 2}} = \sqrt{\frac{35(1.2)^2 + 45(1.0)^2}{78}} = 1.11$$

correct to 2 decimal places (this formula is related to that in Table 8.1).

We now use the same method as above to calculate the standard error we need:

$$\text{s.e.} = \sigma \sqrt{\left(\frac{1}{35} + \frac{1}{45}\right)} = 1.11 \times \sqrt{\left(\frac{1}{35} + \frac{1}{45}\right)} = 0.25$$

and this is what we use to calculate the score used to test our hypothesis.

To test the hypothesis we next calculate the score of our sample-of-one. By the standard method the score is:

$$\frac{\left(\overline{x_M} - \overline{x_W}\right) - (\mu - \mu)}{\text{s.e.}} = \frac{(14 - 11)}{0.25}$$

(using the value for the standard error that we have just found).

Because of the way we have estimated μ, we must deal with this in a different way from the z-scores we have obtained up until now: this score is known as a **t-score**, and the test we are using is an **independent t-test**. In estimating σ we see that we have the number '35 + 45 – 2 = 78' underneath the fraction; this is *the sum of both the sample sizes, less two*, and it is called the number of **degrees of freedom (df)**. So here df = 78 and we call the t-score 't_{78}'; we have:

$$t_{78} = \frac{(14 - 11)}{0.25} = 12$$

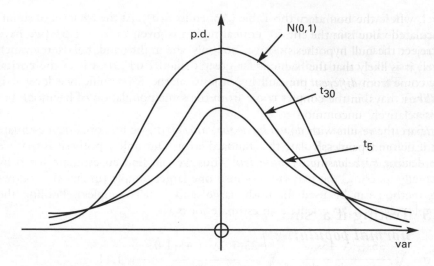

Figure 9.6   The shapes of some t-curves, compared with N(0,1)

A word about t-scores: the individual t-scores indicate points under different curves, and all these **t-curves** are symmetrical about a mean of zero and have a slightly flattened bell shape. However t-curves are *not* standard normal curves. Instead there is a *family* of t-curves: every different number of 'degrees of free-dom' corresponds to a slightly different t-curve (see Figure 9.6), and as the number of degrees of freedom increases so the t-curves gets closer and closer to the shape of the normal curve, $N(0,1^2)$.

For our purposes, any t-curve (here the t_{78}-curve) can be used in the same way as the standard normal curve. At a given significance level a critical region is defined; if the t-score lies within the critical region we *reject* the null hypoth-esis ('the two samples are unlikely to come from the same population'), and if not we *accept* the null hypothesis ('the two samples probably come from the same population').

The Table for t-scores (see Appendix 5(c)) is read differently from the Tables for z-scores. We read down the first column to reach the number of degrees of freedom we are dealing with (or the number just less than it), then along that row. The Table gives us the t-score ('t_U') which bounds the right-hand critical region under the curve, depending on whether we are applying a two-tailed test or a one-tailed test, at a 5% or 1% level of significance. (Where appropriate, we get 't_L', the limit of the left-hand critical region, by symmetry.) In our example on haemoglobin levels, we calculated $t_{78} = 12$, with 78 degrees of freedom. The Table tells us that, when df = 78 and we are testing at the 5% significance level, then the boundary of the critical region is 't = 1.671'. (We use a 'one-tailed test' here because – as we have arranged it – the t-score must be positive; see Section 9.6.) Obviously, our calculated value far exceeds the value from the Table, so it most definitely is in the critical region. Applying our test at the 1% significance level, where the boundary of the critical region is 't = 2.390' we see that the calculated value is in the critical region at this level also. Thus we have evidence to reject the null hypothesis: at the 5% level of significance (or even at the 1% level) it is likely that the haemoglobin levels of the men and the women actually come from *different* populations.

These days, in the context of SPSS and other statistical computer packages, it is relatively uncommon to calculate t-values (or z-values) 'by hand', and compare the results with tabulated values. Computer packages do all this automatically and painlessly – they also provide results with more precision and more accuracy, releasing us to make judgements and draw conclusions.

9.5 Testing if a 'small' sample comes from a *known normal population*

We must be very clear that the methods used in Section 9.3 and Section 9.4 (σ known) depend on the fact that we have 'large' samples. Whenever we are dealing with **small samples** (of sample size 30 or less) taken from a normally distributed population then we adapt our techniques: *we must use the t-score* (not the z-score).

Suppose we wish to find whether it is probable that a small sample of six women (n = 6) have blood pressures which come from the normal population; the population mean for systolic blood pressure is known to be μ = 125 mmHg. The test we use is the **one sample t-test**, based on the sample mean. We calculate the sample mean to be 116 mmHg (say), and the possibility exists that these

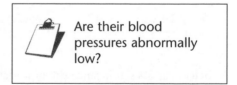

Are their blood pressures abnormally low?

six women come from a genetic grouping whose overall blood pressures are lower than normal. The null hypothesis is that the sample group really *does* come from the normal population, and as a consequence our sample mean *does* belong to 'the distribution of sample means' (see Section 8.3). Since we have the mean of our sample, $\bar{x}$ = 116, we use this as our sample-of-one. Once we decide which level of significance to apply, our working mirrors that in Section 9.3.

If we know the standard deviation of the population, suppose that σ = 12, then we use this to estimate the standard error of the distribution of the sample means:

$$\text{s.e.} = \frac{\sigma}{\sqrt{n}} = \frac{12}{\sqrt{6}} = 4.90$$

From this we obtain the t-score for $\bar{x}$ = 116, the sample-of-one:

$$t_5 = \frac{\bar{x} - \mu}{\left(\dfrac{\sigma}{\sqrt{n}}\right)} = \frac{116 - 125}{4.90} = \frac{-9}{4.90} = -1.84$$

The number of degrees of freedom is '5', which is *the sample size less one*. We use this t-score, $t_5 = -1.84$, to test our hypothesis. The Table in Appendix 5(c) tells us that with df = 5, at the 5% level of significance, for a one-tailed test, the boundary of the critical region is '$t_L = -2.015$' (we are only interested in the left-hand tail). The calculated t-score does not lie in the critical region, so we accept the null hypothesis ('the sample probably does come from the normal population').

If we do not know the standard deviation of the population, then as in Section 9.3, we can estimate for the standard error using the sample's standard deviation, which we take to be s = 10 (say):

$$\text{s.e.} = \frac{s}{\sqrt{n-1}} = \frac{10}{\sqrt{5}} = 4.47$$

There are still 5 degrees of freedom (*the size of the sample less one*), so from this we obtain the t-score:

$$t_5 = \frac{\bar{x} - \mu}{\left(\dfrac{10}{\sqrt{5}}\right)} = \frac{116 - 125}{4.47} = \frac{-9}{4.47} = -2.013$$

As before, at 5% significance the boundary of the critical region is '$t_L = -2.015$' (we are only interested in the left-hand tail). Thus we see again that our t-score does not lie in the critical region, so we accept the null hypothesis ('the sample probably does come from the normal population').

Whether we know the value of σ or not, our calculations do not give us the evidence to say that these six women come from a grouping with recognisably lower blood pressures than normal.

9.6 Two-tailed tests and one-tailed tests

In many of the previous sections we have used 'two-tailed tests' for testing hypotheses. The critical region is in the *two tails* – areas symmetrically placed at the far left and far right under the curve (see Figure 9.7). The reason is that many hypotheses lead us to testing whether a sample-of-one has a score in the critical region, not 'which end' of the critical region it may lie in. For example, in most cases our null hypothesis is that 'this sample belongs to a given population' and

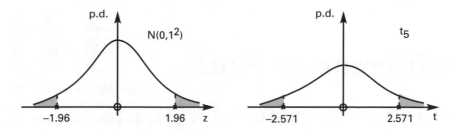

Figure 9.7 5% critical region with two tails, $N(0,1^2)$ and t_5

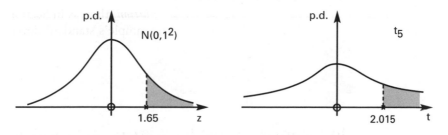

Figure 9.8 5% critical region in right-hand tail, $N(0,1^2)$ and t_5

the alternative hypothesis is merely that 'it does not' – without any preconceived expectation that when the alternative hypothesis applies the sample might be 'extreme' at one end of the range rather than at the other. When we use SPSS all tests are two-tailed.

While two-tailed tests are more common in practice, there are some occasions when a **one-tailed test** can be used, as we have seen. This depends very much on the design of our enquiry, and whether our questioning is 'evenhanded'. As an example of where the expectation is *not* even handed, we consider a null hypothesis that a given group of patients have a *usual* pain threshold, with the alternative hypothesis that this group has an *above average* pain threshold. We use the method of Section 9.3 or Section 9.5, but we would only consider the z-score (or t-score) of the sample-of-one to be in the critical region if it is in the *right-hand tail*, which is the *highest 5%* of the area, at the 5% significance level (see Figure 9.8).

Different or Not? **10**

— using t-scores and ANOVA to compare samples, and techniques to judge clinical significance

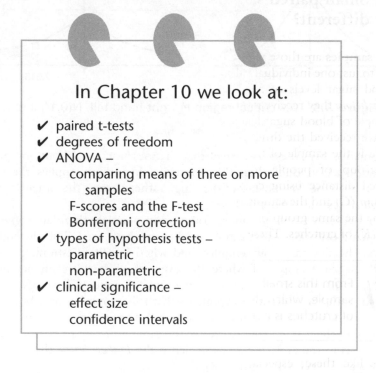

In Chapter 10 we look at:

- ✔ paired t-tests
- ✔ degrees of freedom
- ✔ ANOVA –
  - comparing means of three or more
    samples
  - F-scores and the F-test
  - Bonferroni correction
- ✔ types of hypothesis tests –
  - parametric
  - non-parametric
- ✔ clinical significance –
  - effect size
  - confidence intervals

There are many clinical situations where we wish to test very specific hypotheses, sometimes when we are working with *small samples* (data from groups of 30 or fewer people). An obvious case is when we wish to evaluate the efficacy of some treatment: dealing with the *same group* of people we obtain *two sets of sample data*, from before and after the treatment. Here both the samples have the same number of values, and the values can be 'paired', depending on which patient they relate to. We can easily envisage yet other occasions when we might need to compare *more than two* groups of patients.

To deal with the above situations we show how we use a t-test for 'pairs' and, since t-tests alone are inefficient when we have more than two samples, we introduce the technique known as **ANOVA**.

By any one of the methods discussed in this book we may decide that samples *are* different because their sample means are, statistically, 'significantly different'. But is the difference we see *clinically significant*? In many cases, before we make medical changes or take other action on behalf of patients, it is *essential* that we also consider the relative sizes of the effects recorded compared with the sample means.

10.1 Small paired samples: are they significantly different?

Paired samples are those where each individual value in one sample is directly related to just one individual value in the other sample. One example is a sample of blood sugar levels of a group of patients *before* they receive a drug and the sample of blood sugar levels *after* they have received the drug. Another example is the sample of times taken by a group of people to walk a measured distance using crutches of *one design (C)* and the sample of times

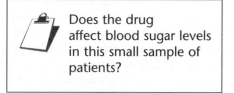

Does the drug affect blood sugar levels in this small sample of patients?

taken by the same group of people to walk the same distance using a *different design (K)* of crutches. These are both cases where we are considering just one group of people: the two samples represent measurements taken on two different occasions. It is obvious that the samples are 'paired': each person in the group generates one value in each.

From this small sample, which design of crutches is better?

How do we begin to compare samples like these, especially when the number of individuals might be 'small'? How can we investigate for significant differences between the samples? We may wish to test whether one design of crutch is an improvement on the other, but differences in the agility of the individuals concerned might 'swamp' any recorded difference in their use of the two sets of crutches. Thus while we could just compare the mean values of the two sets of readings, those figures alone might not be very informative – because the variation between individuals might be far larger than any difference between the means.

So, instead of calculating separate sample means, we actively use the fact that the samples' values are paired: we calculate *the numerical difference* between each pair of related values. In our first example, for each patient we calculate:

'blood sugar level *before* drug given' minus 'blood sugar level *after* drug given';

and in our second example, for each person we calculate:

'time to walk using *C crutches*' minus 'time to walk using *K crutches*'.

The number of items (n) in this list of numerical differences is the same as the number of values in each of the original samples. It is important that we do the subtractions the 'same way round' for each individual, so that every time it is ' "value before" minus "value after" ', or ' "time with C" minus "time with K" '. Thus for each patient we get a number, d, where:

d = first measurement – second measurement

and it is quite acceptable to get negative numbers in this process.

We are looking for any significant differences between the original samples, so we take as our null hypothesis that 'the samples are effectively indistinguishable'. In other words our null hypotheses might be 'the levels of blood sugar are unchanged by the drug' or 'neither type of crutch gives an advantage over the other'. We now take the list of numerical differences obtained by subtraction (the set of 'd' values, as above) as a sample in its own right, and calculate the sample mean, $\bar{d}$. If the drug has no effect, or each type of crutch gives no advantage, then we expect the value of $\bar{d}$ to be very small and the population mean of all possible 'd s' (which we here call $\bar{D}$) to be zero.

We now use t-scores in a third type of hypothesis test, **a paired t-test** (called sometimes a **related t-test**, or a **dependent t-test**). If we assume that the distribution of the population of 'd s' is normal, then the distribution of sample means, from which $\bar{d}$ comes, is also normal – so we test our hypothesis using a method like that in Section 9.5. By the null hypothesis the population mean is zero, that is '$\bar{D} = 0$', and it is usual to test at a 5% significance level.

Having calculated the sample mean, $\bar{d}$, we also determine the sample standard deviation, s_d. Since we do not know the standard deviation of the population, we estimate the standard error of the sample means from this sample standard deviation:

$$\text{s.e.} = \frac{s_d}{\sqrt{n-1}}$$

(The number 'n – 1' is the number of degrees of freedom; it is the *original number of people/patients, less one*). We calculate the t-score for $\bar{d}$ by:

$$t_{n-1} = \frac{\bar{d} - \bar{D}}{s.e.}$$

and since '$\bar{D} = 0$' by our hypothesis we have:

$$t_{n-1} = \frac{\bar{d}}{s.e.}$$

Using Statistical Tables (see Appendix 5(c)) we test whether this t-score lies in the critical region (at 5% significance). If it *does*, we *reject the null hypothesis*, and deduce that there probably *is* some significant difference between the original two samples: that is, the drug *does* have an effect on blood sugar levels, or there *is* some advantage in one or other of the two types of crutches. Otherwise, we accept the null hypothesis: at the 5% level there is no significant difference detected.

10.2 Degrees of freedom

In all three of the types of t-tests – independent t-tests, one sample t-tests and now paired t-tests – we have met the term **degrees of freedom** (Sections 9.4, 9.5 and 10.1). This is an important concept that we shall meet several times more in the sections and chapters that follow. As with many other ideas, we do not need to understand everything about degrees of freedom before we use them: it is often possible to 'follow the rules' without necessarily understanding the theory in depth. However, since this is an important concept we now discuss a bit about where it comes from.

The first time we implicitly met degrees of freedom was in Section 8.2, looking at an unbiased estimator for the variance of a population. From a sample of size 'n' with variance 's^2', we estimated the population variance by:

$$\sigma^2 \approx \left(\frac{n}{n-1} \right) s^2$$

Then in Section 8.5 we had the estimate for the standard error:

$$s.e. \approx \frac{s}{\sqrt{n-1}}$$

The 'n – 1' under both of these fractions is the number of *degrees of freedom*; in these cases we see that it is *the sample size less one.*

In general terms, the number of degrees of freedom refers to the number of *independent values* in our sample. The calculation of a sample mean by the formula:

$$\bar{x} = \frac{\Sigma x}{n}$$

involves 'n' values and so 'n' degrees of freedom. So why is the number of degrees of freedom reduced from 'n' to 'n – 1' when we are dealing with parameters that are *estimated*?

Suppose we did *not* have to estimate the population parameters, because we could calculate them directly. Using the methods of Sections 5.2 and 5.3, if there are 'n' values of the variable 'x' in the population then the population mean is:

$$\mu = \frac{\Sigma x}{n}$$

and the population variance is:

$$\sigma^2 = \frac{\Sigma(x - \mu)^2}{n}$$

The 'n' under both of these fractions is the number of independent values we have, so here the number of degrees of freedom is 'n'.

But if we are *unable* to calculate μ directly we must estimate it using the value $\bar{x}$ (calculated from a sample of size 'n'). In this case we estimate the population variance by:

$$\sigma^2 \approx \frac{\Sigma(x - \bar{x})^2}{n} \times \frac{n}{n - 1}$$

(remembering that we must 'scale up' by:

$$\frac{n}{n - 1}$$

(see Section 8.2) because a variance based on only a sample underestimates the true value for the population). Thus we obtain an estimate for the population variance:

$$\sigma^2 \approx \frac{\Sigma(x - \bar{x})^2}{n - 1}$$

Here we no longer have 'n' *independent* values for the variable 'x'. While we certainly do have 'n' values for 'x' in the sample, we also know their mean, so the 'xs' are connected by:

$$\bar{x} = \frac{\Sigma x}{n}$$

that is:

$$\Sigma x = n\,\bar{x}$$

From this, we see that whenever we know the values of all-but-one of the 'xs' we can *calculate* the last value of 'x' – *because we know their sample mean*. Thus only 'n − 1' of the 'xs' are truly 'independent'; the number of degrees of freedom is 'n − 1' which is the number underneath the fraction in the above formula for σ^2.

This briefly is why, when we are dealing with an *estimated population mean*, the calculation of the population variance involves *'sample size less one'* degrees of freedom.

The concept of degrees of freedom is necessary in the t-tests of Sections 9.4, 9.5 and 10.1 because the population means and variances are estimated, in ways similar to those described above. Degrees of freedom are also used in the following sections of this chapter, and in the techniques introduced in Chapters 11 and 13.

10.3 Comparing more than two samples at a time – ANOVA

In previous sections we have considered cases where we wished to compare two samples at a time, but it is easy to think of situations where we might wish to compare *more than two* samples. For example, we could take measurements from two (or more) groups of patients who have been offered different treatments, and compare these with a **control group**, who were offered no treatment, or a standardised treatment.

When comparing three or more groups like this, looking for any significant differences, it would be possible – but extremely tedious and inefficient – to apply independent t-tests repeatedly from the outset, comparing the samples two-at-a-time. (We must be clear: usually these are *not* 'paired samples'.) For three samples taken two-at-a-time there would be three comparisons; for four samples taken two-at-a-time there would be six comparisons; five samples would need ten comparisons and six samples would need fifteen comparisons. The number of calculations needed rises alarmingly! – this is *not* a preferred method.

To deal with the comparison of more than two samples in a single test we need a technique that takes into account the statistical features (means, standard deviations, etc.) of all the samples. In addition, as with the paired t-test, we need this test to be able to discriminate between 'the variation between individuals within a sample' and 'the variation between sample means'. The test we use, called **ANOVA** (the acronym for **AN**alysis **O**f **VA**riance), does a task that is, broadly speaking, similar to that of the independent t-test: indeed, if we are comparing just two samples, then ANOVA and the t-test give the same result. The results from ANOVA are valid so long as the samples are independent and they come from normal populations.

Suppose, for example, that we have data from three different samples, A, B and C: these are three groups of patients who have received different treatments. If there are n individuals in each group, then we calculate the three sample means, $\overline{x_A}$, $\overline{x_B}$, $\overline{x_C}$; in general they will *not* be identical. We must decide whether the samples are 'essentially the same': that it is likely that they come from the same population (with any differences due merely to random variation within the samples). Alternatively, if they come from different populations, then any differences between them are likely to be due to the different treatments. This analysis is a **one-way analysis of variance**, with *one* possible element of imposed variation. We use the *variances* (see Section 5.3) of the samples for a specific technical reason: unlike standard deviations, *variances can be added and subtracted*.

> Three groups of patients, three different treatments: are the outcomes different or essentially the same?

Using the ANOVA technique we test the (null) hypothesis that the different treatments have caused no significantly different effects, that is, all the three samples come from the same population. The calculations involve us in using rather different methods to obtain *two estimates* for the variance of this population. The first method depends on the measurements of the variance *within* each sample; we call it the **within-sample variation**. This is '*estimate (1)*' and it tells us about the amount of variability due to random variations in the individuals *in each sample*. The second method gives us an estimate for the population variance based on the distribution of the sample means. This is '*estimate (2)*', called the **between-sample variation**, and it tells us about the variability *between the sample means* – which would indicate any variability introduced by the treatments.

Our null hypothesis is that the treatments have caused no significantly different effects, in which case *both* estimates for the variance will refer to the *same* population variance. The closer the two estimates are, the more likely it is that the samples come from the same population: the treatments have had no significant effects.

To test the null hypothesis we calculate the **F-score** for the two estimates for variance. The F-score of the estimates is their ratio (always arranged so that the *larger* estimate is on the *top* of the fraction):

$$F = \frac{estimate(1)}{estimate(2)} \text{ (or it might be } \frac{estimate(2)}{estimate(1)} \text{)}$$

As we have mentioned, we are likely to accept the null hypothesis when these two estimates are very close, and in this case their ratio (the above fraction) will be very close to 'one'. When the value of the ratio gets larger, and further away from 'one', then we are more likely to reject the null hypothesis and conclude that one of the treatments *has* made a significant difference. To decide whether the F-score is significant, we apply the **F-test** (sometimes called the **variance ratio test**). The critical values of F are obtained from Tables (see Appendix 5(g)).

We now look briefly at the type of calculations involved in finding an F-score. We are testing the hypothesis that the three samples above come from the same population and, finally, we shall illustrate the method using some simple numbers.

For the *within-sample variation*, we estimate the population variance (σ^2) using the information from each separate sample in turn. First, taking the values in sample A, we find an estimate for the population variance based on the expression we found in Section 10.2:

$$\sigma^2 = \frac{\Sigma(x - \overline{x_A})^2}{n - 1}$$

Next we do exactly the same for sample B and sample C. We then mentally combine the three samples, so we add together the three formulae (details are shown in Appendix 4(a)). This gives us the overall *within-sample* estimate for the population variance σ^2:

$$\sigma^2 = \frac{\Sigma(x - \overline{x_A})^2 + \Sigma(x - \overline{x_B})^2 + \Sigma(x - \overline{x_C})^2}{3(n - 1)} \qquad (\textit{this is 'estimate (1)'})$$

Here the number '3(n – 1)' is the number of degrees of freedom; it is *'the number of samples' times 'sample size less one'*. The reason for this is similar to that discussed in Section 10.2 above.

We base the estimate for the *between-sample variation* on the relationship between the population variance (unknown in this case) and the variance of sample means. Using Table 8.1, where the population variance is σ^2 and the sample size is 'n', the estimate for the variance of the sample means (= the square of the standard error) is given by:

$$\text{variance of sample means} = \frac{\sigma^2}{n}$$

But we can estimate the variance of sample means by a more direct calculation (see Table 5.3) once we have found $\bar{X}$, the overall mean obtained from mentally combining the three samples. This allows us to calculate the *between-sample* estimate for the population variance (details are shown in Appendix 4(b)). The overall *between-sample* estimate for the population variance σ^2 is:

$$\sigma^2 = \frac{n\Sigma\,(\bar{x} - \bar{X})^2}{3 - 1} \qquad (\textit{this is 'estimate (2)'})$$

The number '3 – 1' (= 2) is the number of degrees of freedom; it is *'the number of samples less one'* (the reasoning is again similar to that discussed in Section 10.2).

Once we have these two estimates, we obtain the F-score by calculating their ratio, putting the larger estimate on the top of the fraction; let us assume that the calculations we are dealing with yield F = 4.5. Before we can use the Table in Appendix 5(g) to find whether this score is 'significant' (at the 5% significance level, say), we need *both* of the degrees of freedom we have calculated. Suppose we are dealing with three groups of patients and 41 patients in each group, then we have three samples and the sample size is n = 41. Thus in 'estimate (1)' the number of degrees of freedom is:

$$3(n - 1) = 3(41 - 1) = 3 \times 40 = 120$$

and we write 'df1 = 120'. In 'estimate (2)' the number of degrees of freedom is:

$$3 - 1 = 2 \text{ (as above)}$$

and so we write 'df2 = 2'. For a result which is significant at the 5% level we look in the first Table of Appendix 5(g): we read down the first column until we reach 'df1 = 120', then along that row until we are beneath the value 'df2 = 2'. We see that the entry in the Table is '3.07'. Clearly, our calculated value of 'F = 4.5' is *larger than* this value in the table, so we have a 'significant' result. We thus reject the null hypothesis and deduce that (at 5% significance) it is likely that not all our three samples come from the same population. In other words, we can conclude that at least one of the treatments *has* made a significant difference.

(If we repeat this test at the 1% significance level, we see that the tabulated value in the second Table of Appendix 5(g) is '4.79'. Since our calculated value, 'F = 4.5', is *less than* this, at the 1% significance level we do *not* have a significant result so we would *not* reject the null hypothesis at this level.)

ANOVA methods are very important and have considerable practical use in the analysis of research data. The calculations sketched out above can, of course, become very involved and tedious. Most work on 'real' examples is done using computer software.

If ANOVA gives a 'significant' result, then at least one of the samples is significantly different from the others. To test which it might be we must do further work, probably by applying an independent t-test to each pair of samples. When multiple comparison tests are carried out in a situation like this – after ANOVA has indicated 'significant' – then the risk of a type I error (see Section 7.5) is magnified. The consequence of a type I error in this case is that a difference is identified erroneously, where none exists in fact. When we have *many* tests, then the possibility of one of them showing a 'significant difference' due to just random chance increases enormously. Thus to keep the *overall* risk of a type I error at 5% (say), we apply the **Bonferroni correction** to all the subsequent comparison tests. This involves *reducing* the level of significance used in all the subsequent tests: at each test we do not use 5% significance but we apply the significance level of:

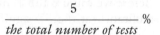

$$\frac{5}{\text{the total number of tests}}\%$$

In the case above we have three samples and comparing these in pairs involves three tests – so for these tests we use a significance level of $\frac{5}{3}$% which is approximately 1.7%. (If we had started with four samples then comparing them in pairs involves six tests, and so for each one we would use a significance level of $\frac{5}{6}$%, about 0.83; and so on.)

10.4 Other tests for differences between samples

In comparing samples so that we can compare groups of people, all the hypothesis tests so far discussed involve 'parameters' (the summary values for *populations* like mean, variance and standard deviation); they are called **parametric tests**. To use these parameters we have needed to assume that we are dealing with very large samples and/or that the data are normally distributed; in health related research

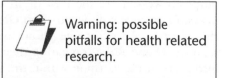

Warning: possible pitfalls for health related research.

these assumptions may, or may not be, valid. In addition, to avoid bias, the statistical tests demand that samples are selected at random: in health related research they rarely are.

There is another category of hypothesis tests altogether called **non-parametric tests**, where samples can be compared without us making assumptions about the distribution of the populations or calculating any parameters. These are useful in dealing with small samples especially where the level of measurement used in the study is ordinal, so that the data values are merely ranked (they are not necessarily equidistant as in interval measure, still less is there necessarily an 'intrinsic zero' as in ratio measure). Where non-parametric tests can be used they often allow for stronger conclusions.

Non-parametric tests include the **chi-squared test** (see Chapter 11), **Spearman's rank-correlation test** (see Section 12.6), the **sign test**, the **Wilcoxon test**, the **Kruskal-Wallis test** and the **Mann-Whitney U test**. In general terms we can say that every parametric test has a non-parametric equivalent. For example, the Mann-Whitney U test can be used to test whether the difference between two sets of ranked data is statistically significantly: it is the non-parametric equivalent of the t-test. If we are interested in comparing more than two sets of ranked data then the appropriate test is the Kruskal-Wallis test, the non-parametric equivalent of ANOVA.

Over many years there has been much debate about the relative merits of the two types of tests. It was often cautioned that if there was any doubt about the choice then a non-parametric test should be used. However, for most purposes the result obtained is independent of the test used. Here we shall not look at any non-parametric tests except as mentioned above.

10.5 Deciding on clinically important differences: effect size

Even if our calculations tell us that there is a significant difference (at the 5% level, say) between two sample means, we cannot sensibly proceed to make clinical decisions without taking other matters into account.

If sample sizes are very large, a 'small' overall difference between means might show up as statistically significant, but the *actual* difference might be *so small* as to be *clinically insignificant*. On the other hand, especially when sample sizes are small, a clinically important difference might not appear as statistically significant. To help us interpret these differences for practical purposes we can use the idea of an **effect size**: decisions in clinical practice depend not merely on whether an effect has been detected, but on how large the effect is. An effect size allows us to gauge the difference between two samples, Q and R, by comparing their sample means ($\overline{x_Q}$ and $\overline{x_R}$) while taking into account the variation within the samples (their standard deviations are s_Q and s_R respectively).

The calculation for 'effect size' is unsophisticated, quick and simple. We start by finding s_p, an **'averaged' standard deviation** for the samples. This is obtained from the 'average' of the two sample variances:

$$s_p^2 = \tfrac{1}{2}(s_Q^2 + s_R^2)$$

$$\text{so } s_p = \sqrt{\frac{s_Q{}^2 + s_R{}^2}{2}}$$

Then we find the **effect size**, ES, by:

$$ES = \frac{\overline{x_Q} - \overline{x_R}}{s_p}$$

To illustrate the issue of 'effect size', we imagine we are investigating the effect of relaxation therapy on the blood pressure of hypertensive patients. The patients are divided into two groups of equal size, Q and R, one of which (R) receives the relaxation therapy. After a month each patient's blood pressure is recorded, and the mean blood pressure for each group is calculated. Suppose the sample mean for group (R) is 5 mmHg lower than the sample mean for the control group (Q): can we say that this justifies the staff-time and expenses in providing the therapy?

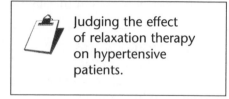

Judging the effect of relaxation therapy on hypertensive patients.

If the same exercise is carried out the following year with different groups of patients, suppose we find that the sample mean for the group (RR) is 8 mmHg lower than the sample mean for the control group (QQ). On the face of things this provides a greater justification for providing the therapy. However, calculations of the effect size may indicate otherwise, as we now show.

To investigate these effect of the relaxation therapy, we can suppose that the 'pooled' standard deviation for the set of blood pressures (the first time) is 10 mmHg. Then we have:

$$ES = \frac{5}{10} = 0.5$$

After a year (the second time), suppose the (pooled) standard deviation is 18 mmHg, then we have:

$$ES = \frac{8}{18} = 0.44$$

Whether or not the individual differences are statistically significant, the difference of 8 mmHg actually represents a *smaller* effect size than the difference of 5 mmHg.

Effect size can be a useful guide for decision making, but the information it provides is limited; it is generally considered to be unsafe to determine clinical significance by relying only on this.

10.6 Deciding on clinically important differences: confidence intervals

Of more use in helping us to decide on the clinical significance of data is the idea of the *confidence interval*, met in Chapter 8. This gives us more precise values to compare, which we may use to justify or decide against clinical intervention.

To illustrate the value of this technique, suppose that we are still investigating the effect of relaxation therapy on hypertensive patients, as we considered above. We use the data from both the samples, (Q) and (R) to calculate the two sample means, ($\overline{x_Q}$ and $\overline{x_R}$), and the two sample standard deviations (s_Q and s_R). From these figures we calculate the confidence interval (typically at 95%) for the value of the (population) mean of the difference between these means. When we know the *size* of this interval then clinical knowledge and experience allows us to make considered judgements concerning the possible effectiveness of this relaxation therapy. Suppose, for example, the 95% confidence interval for the difference in the mean blood pressures between the two groups of patients is from 0.2 mmHg to 1.3 mmHg. At most, this represents a *very small drop* in blood pressure, one unlikely to have any impact on a hypertensive person. Thus the effect of *this* intervention through relaxation therapy is clinically unimpressive. On the other hand, if the 95% confidence interval is from 7.5 mmHg to 10.3 mmHg, then we might judge that a potential improvement could cause a patient to become free of hypertension.

> Another way to judge the effect of relaxation therapy on hypertensive patients.

For calculating confidence intervals, we remember that in Section 8.5 we dealt with the 95% confidence interval for a population mean where we had a *large* sample size. The expression we arrived at is:

$$\overline{x} - (1.96 \times \text{s.e.}) \leq \mu \leq \overline{x} + (1.96 \times \text{s.e.})$$

where $\overline{x}$ is the sample mean that we calculate, μ the population mean and s.e. the standard error of the distribution of sample means. The number '1.96' is the z-score given by Tables because we are looking for the '95%' confidence interval.

If the groups Q and R are *large* samples, then we use the z-score of $z = 1.96$ as before. In the case we are now looking at we replace '$\overline{x}$' by ($\overline{x_Q} - \overline{x_R}$), and the confidence interval is based around $(\overline{\mu_Q} - \overline{\mu_R})$, the mean of the population differences. Since the populations' standard deviations are unknown we obtain an estimate for the standard error of the sampling distribution and then the confidence interval is:

$$(\overline{x_Q} - \overline{x_R}) - (1.96 \times \text{s.e.}) \leq (\overline{\mu_Q} - \overline{\mu_R}) \leq (\overline{x_Q} - \overline{x_R}) + (1.96 \times \text{s.e.})$$

The three different types of t-tests can also be involved in finding confidence limits, as we indicate below.

If we have two samples that we assume come from the same normal population, then we apply the idea of confidence limits by using t-scores (as in Section 9.4 'σ unknown'). We look at the difference between the sample means and we estimate the standard error; then, depending on the number of degrees of freedom (the sum of the sample sizes less two), the Table (Appendix 5(c)) give us the appropriate t-score (we can call this t*) corresponding to the 95% confidence limits. The confidence interval is:

$$(\overline{x_Q} - \overline{x_R}) - (\text{t*} \times \text{s.e.}) \leq (\overline{\mu_Q} - \overline{\mu_R}) \leq (\overline{x_Q} - \overline{x_R}) + (\text{t*} \times \text{s.e.})$$

This method also works to obtain a confidence interval for a population mean (μ) if we have a single small sample (size n, mean $\bar{x}$ and standard deviation s from which we estimate the standard error as in Section 9.5). In this case the confidence interval for the mean of the normal population is:

$$\bar{x} - (\text{t*} \times \text{s.e.}) \leq \mu \leq \bar{x} + (\text{t*} \times \text{s.e.})$$

We can also use the same method to find the confidence interval for the mean of numerical differences (as in the paired t-test, Section 10.1). The confidence interval in this case is:

$$\bar{d} - (\text{t*} \times \text{s.e.}) \leq \overline{D} \leq \bar{d} + (\text{t*} \times \text{s.e.})$$

So we can use data from a sample to give information about the *confidence interval of the mean* of a population. Knowing this it is often possible to apply clinical knowledge and judgement to decide whether perceived differences are *really clinically significant.*

The Significance of Proportions

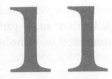

– *using contingency tables and the chi-squared (χ^2) test to compare proportions*

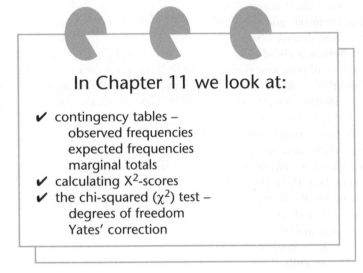

In Chapter 11 we look at:

✔ contingency tables –
    observed frequencies
    expected frequencies
    marginal totals
✔ calculating X^2-scores
✔ the chi-squared (χ^2) test –
    degrees of freedom
    Yates' correction

In nursing and other areas of healthcare, we are often able to measure a variable at *nominal level only*. There are many situations where this lowest level of measurement is the only one possible: for example a patient might be recorded as 'given treatment' or 'not given treatment', they might be 'better' or 'worse', and – ultimately – they will be 'alive' or 'dead'. But all our consideration until now has been given to cases where variables are measured *above* nominal level – sometimes at interval or ratio level, but always at least at ordinal level. In this chapter we look at some tools for dealing with nominal variables and in particular at a *non-parametric test* which helps us make judgements when all the variables are measured at nominal level only. We shall test to see whether it is likely that such variables are essentially unrelated, or alternatively, perhaps connected in some way.

11.1 Contingency tables

A good example of a case study where variables are measured at nominal level is where we take a group of people, some of whom smoke cigarettes, and determine which of them suffer from chest disease. Some, but not all, of the smokers will suffer from chest disease; not all of the non-smokers are free from chest disease. The group can be classified in two different ways: either as 'smokers' and 'non-smokers', or as 'suffering from a chest disease' and 'not suffering from a chest disease'. We see that *everyone* in the group can be classified by both criteria, and everyone falls into one of four classes: 'smoking and suffering a chest disease', 'smoking and *not* suffering a chest disease', '*not* smoking and suffering a chest disease' and '*not* smoking and *not* suffering a chest disease'. We shall compare the *proportions* of people in these classes.

> Is smoking connected with chest disease?

To make this example easy to follow, we use 'easy' numbers to start with. Suppose we initially have a group of 100 people, of whom 50 are smokers. We record that 31 of the smokers and 19 of the non-smokers suffer from chest disease. We immediately see that more of the smokers than the non-smokers suffer from chest disease, but can we deduce more from these numbers? It might be that the smokers really are more susceptible to chest disease than the non-smokers. But 19 of the smokers *do not* suffer from chest disease, and 19 of the non-smokers *do*, so how can we decide whether these numbers may have come about other than by chance?

The first step in making sense of these numbers, and in analysing them, is to present them in a **contingency table**. A contingency table is a rectangular array of boxes or **cells**. Each **column of cells** indicates one classification of the group considered ('smoking/non-smoking' in our example), while each **row of cells** indicates the second classification (here 'with/without chest disease'). In Table 11.1 we show the data in this case. This is a '2 × 2' contingency table, with 2 rows and 2 columns, and we label the four cells (a), (b), (c) and (d) as shown.

Table 11.1 Contingency table for smoking and chest disease

	Smoking		*Non-smoking*	
With chest disease	(a)	31	(b)	19
Without chest disease	(c)	19	(d)	31

Table 11.2 Augmented contingency table (observed frequencies) showing marginal totals

Observed frequencies	Smoking		Non-smoking		Row totals
With chest disease	(a)	31	(b)	19	50
Without chest disease	(c)	19	(d)	31	50
Column totals		50		50	Grand total = 100

We see that every individual in the group can be allocated to precisely one of the cells. In allocating numbers to the cells we count how many individuals belong to the different categories. For example, there are 31 people who are in the 'smoking' category *and also* in the 'with chest disease' category; thus we put '31' in cell (a). The other three cells are filled similarly. These numbers are called the **observed frequencies**.

We next augment the table with an extra column and an extra row where we place the **marginal totals**, as shown in Table 11.2.

The marginal totals are the row totals and the column totals. The first column includes all the people in the category 'smoker', thus the column total is '50' which we get by adding the contents of cells (a) and (c). Similarly we add the contents of cells (b) and (d) to get the marginal total of people in the 'non-smoking' category. In the same way we total the cells in each row to obtain the marginal totals for the categories 'with chest disease' and 'without chest disease'. As a check, adding the row totals *always* gives the same answer as adding the column totals: both give '100' in this table, as shown in the bottom right-hand cell. Here '100' is the size of the whole group: it is the **grand total**, the **total frequency** of people in the study.

The second step in analysing these figures is to create the contingency table which we would *expect* to see from our study if 'smoking' and 'chest diseases' were quite **independent** (that is, totally unrelated in any way) – this is our *null hypothesis*. The table (see Table 11.3) has the same marginal totals: the numbers of smokers is unchanged and we would expect equal numbers in each category (the 'smokers' and the 'non-smokers') to develop a chest disease.

We write the **expected frequencies** in the cells. Because the first row contains '50' (that is, 50% of the total) and each column entry contains 50% of the row

Table 11.3 Augmented contingency table for expected frequencies

Expected frequencies	Smoking		Non-smoking		Row totals
With chest disease	(a)	25	(b)	25	50
Without chest disease	(c)	25	(d)	25	50
Column totals		50		50	Grand total = 100

total, cell (a) contains '25'. In this example, every cell contains '25': once the row totals and the column totals are in place, there is no other result possible when we calculate the expected frequencies for the four cells. By comparing these two tables – for observed frequencies and expected frequencies – we shall be able to test whether the variables are (probably) independent (in Sections 11.2 and 11.3 which follow).

How do we create pairs of contingency tables when the data are not *quite* so contrived? In a second case study we might have a grand total of 80 smokers who state that they wish to give up their smoking habit. 50 of these agree to attend a weekly 'Health Education Group (H.E.G.)' where they are supported in their decision and given practical help and advice in stopping smoking; the rest choose

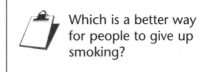

Which is a better way for people to give up smoking?

to follow their own individual course. After three months 32 of those attending the weekly sessions have (still) given up smoking and 12 are smoking fewer cigarettes each day. Of those 'going solo', 14 have stopped smoking and 4 are smoking less. Can we decide whether putting on the Health Education Group is a worthwhile exercise? Are the 'quitting smoking' success rates shown by those who attended it *significantly* better than the 'solo' group's?

Table 11.4 shows the contingency table for these observed frequencies. From the six figures we are given (shown circled) we can easily find the contents of all the other cells and the marginal totals.

We would like to use these figures to find how likely it is that the resources put into the Health Education Group have been effectively used. So we construct a second contingency table (Table 11.5) of expected frequencies, *working just from the marginal totals.*

The expected frequencies we want are the *theoretical* ones, based just on the proportions given by the marginal totals. By our null hypothesis we assume that the 'success rates' are independent of whether an individual receives support or not.

To calculate the expected frequency for cell (a), we look at the column totals

Table 11.4 Augmented contingency table for giving up smoking – H.E.G. supported or 'solo' (observed frequencies)

Observed frequencies	Given up	Smoking less	No change	Row totals
H.E.G. supported	(a) 32	(b) 12	(c) 6	50
'Solo'	(d) 14	(e) 4	(f) 12	30
Column totals	46	16	18	Grand total = 80

Table 11.5   Augmented contingency table for giving up smoking – H.E.G. supported or 'solo' (expected frequencies)

Expected frequencies	Given up	Smoking less	No change	Row totals
H.E.G. supported	(a)	(b)	(c)	50
'Solo'	(d)	(e)	(f)	30
Column totals	46	16	18	Grand total = 80

and see that, overall, $^{46}/_{80}$ths of the whole group have given up smoking. But from the row totals we see that 50 of the group attend the H.E.G., so the *expected* frequency of those who have given up smoking who attend the H.E.G. is:

$$\frac{46}{80} \times 50 = 28.75$$

For cell (b) we calculate $^{16}/_{80}$ths of the 50 people who attend the H.E.G.: the *expected* frequency of those smoking less who attend the H.E.G. is:

$$\frac{16}{80} \times 50 = 10$$

Similarly, the number for cell (c) is:

$$\frac{18}{80} \times 50 = 11.25$$

The calculations for the second row are these: the number for cell (d) is:

$$\frac{46}{80} \times 30 = 17.25$$

the number for cell (e) is:

$$\frac{16}{80} \times 30 = 6$$

and the number for cell (f) is:

Table 11.6   Augmented contingency table for giving up smoking – H.E.G. supported or 'solo' (expected frequencies)

Expected frequencies	Given up	Smoking less	No change	Row totals
H.E.G. supported	(a) 28.75	(b) 10	(c) 11.25	50
'Solo'	(d) 17.25	(e) 6	(f) 6.75	30
Column totals	46	16	18	Grand total = 80

$$\frac{18}{80} \times 30 = 6.75$$

Put briefly, for each cell we obtain the expected frequency by:

$$\text{expected frequency} = \frac{\text{column total} \times \text{row total}}{\text{grand total}}$$

When we put all these expected frequencies into the contingency table (see Table 11.6), we can check that all the row totals and column totals do indeed add up correctly (they do!).

11.2   Calculating the χ^2-score for a contingency table

As shown above, a contingency table allows us to record, in a concise manner, data obtained by categorising a sample according to two different criteria.

In our first case study each variable, measured at a nominal level, yields just two categories. For the variable 'smoking status' we have 'smoker/non-smoker' and for the variable 'health indicator' we have 'suffers from/does not suffer from chest disease'. Thus our first case study gives a '2 × 2' contingency table (we do *not* include the marginal cells when describing the size of the table).

In our second case study there are three categories for the variable 'smoking status', namely 'given up smoking/smoking less/no change'; and two categories for the variable 'method of giving up smoking', namely 'H.E.G. supported/solo'. Here we have a '2 × 3' contingency tables (we count 'the number of rows' × 'the number of columns' – in that order). In general, '2 × 2', '2 × 3', '3 × 2', '3 × 3' and other size contingency tables are all common, depending on how many interventions and outcomes are of interest.

Contingency tables allow us to analyse data as well as recording it. Specifically, they allow us to test the null hypothesis that the two variables are independent; in the cases above this is the same as testing that the outcomes occur by chance, not influenced by the interventions. To test this null hypothesis we calculate the sample statistic called the χ^2-**score** for the pair of contingency tables, that is, for the table of observed frequencies and the corresponding table of expected frequencies. The χ^2-score is based on the numbers in the cells (*not* on the marginal totals). The **symbol** χ^2 uses the Greek letter χ (it is *not* the letter X). χ is written as 'chi' but pronounced like the 'ki' in 'kind'.

For each cell in turn we subtract the expected frequency (E) from the observed frequency (O), square the result and then divide it by the expected frequency. So for each cell we calculate:

$$\frac{(O-E)^2}{E}$$

and then we add all these numbers together: this total is the χ^2-score for the tables. When we have a *small* value for χ^2 then we know that the observed and expected frequencies are 'quite close', so it is likely that the numbers we have gathered have occurred by chance.

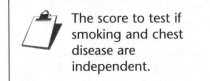
The score to test if smoking and chest disease are independent.

In the first case study of Section 11.1 (investigating whether the status of 'smoker' affected the propensity to chest disease), we use the numbers from the cells in Tables 11.2 and 11.3 to calculate the χ^2-score:

$$\chi^2 = \frac{(31-25)^2}{25} + \frac{(19-25)^2}{25} + \frac{(19-25)^2}{25} + \frac{(31-25)^2}{25}$$

$$= \frac{36}{25} + \frac{36}{25} + \frac{36}{25} + \frac{36}{25} = 5.76$$

For the second case study in Section 11.1 (investigating whether H.E.G. support made a significant contribution to success in quitting smoking), we obtain from Tables 11.4 and 11.6:

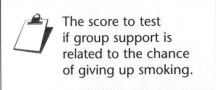
The score to test if group support is related to the chance of giving up smoking.

$$\chi^2 = \frac{(32-28.75)^2}{28.75} + \frac{(12-10)^2}{10} + \frac{(6-11.25)^2}{11.25} + \frac{(14-17.25)^2}{17.25}$$

$$+ \frac{(4-6)^2}{6} + \frac{(12-6.75)^2}{6.75}$$

$$= 0.37 + 0.4 + 2.45 + 0.61 + 0.67 + 4.08$$
$$= 8.58$$

These calculations can be done easily with a calculator; the results are quoted accurate to two places of decimals.

11.3 Applying the chi-squared (χ^2) test for proportions

Once we have calculated the value of the sample statistic χ^2 for the proportions under investigation we can find whether our result is 'significant' (that is, *probably not* merely due to chance) by applying what is known as the **chi-squared test**. We use the Table for χ^2 (see Appendix 5(d)) to determine the significance of our results.

Like the t-test, the chi-squared test depends on us knowing the relevant number of *degrees of freedom* involved. The number of degrees of freedom for a chi-squared test is given by the *size* of the contingency table. The general rule is that the number of degrees of freedom is:

'(number of rows, less one) × (number of columns, less one)'.

In our first case study we use a '2 × 2' table so there is:

$(2 - 1) \times (2 - 1) = 1 \times 1 = 1$ degree of freedom.

Our second case study uses a '2 × 3' table, so we have:

$(2 - 1) \times (3 - 1) = 1 \times 2 = 2$ degrees of freedom.

This rule for degrees of freedom is quite consistent with Section 10.2: the number of degrees of freedom counts how many *independent variables* we have in the system. If we know all the marginal totals, then the number of degrees of freedom corresponds with the number of values which can be independently inserted into the contingency table. For example, freely inserting *just one* value into a cell in a '2 × 2' table (where we know the marginal totals) determines the contents of the other three cells, so they are *dependent* on it; there is *one* degree of freedom in this case. Similarly, freely inserting *just two* independent values into cells in a '2 × 3' table fixes the contents of the other four cells.

In Figure 11.1 we indicate how the shape of the chi-squared distribution changes according to the number of degrees of freedom.

In practical situations most hypothesis testing using the chi-squared test is done with an appropriate computer package, but at this stage we can easily

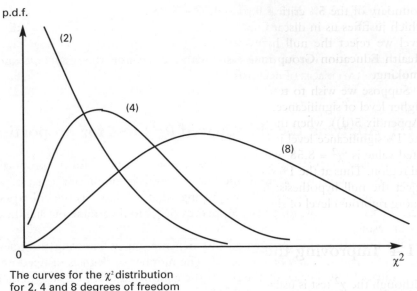

The curves for the χ^2 distribution
for 2, 4 and 8 degrees of freedom
are indicated

Figure 11.1   The shape of the chi-squared distribution

use our Table to determine whether the results of our two case studies are significant.

For our first case study (investigating whether the status of 'smoker' affected the propensity to chest disease) we have '1' degree of freedom and calculated χ^2 = 5.76. The Table in Appendix 5(d) tells us that the critical region at the 5% significance level is bounded by the value 'χ^2 = 3.84'. In this case it is clear that our figure of '5.76' is greater than '3.84', thus it *is* in the critical region and so we have reason to discard the null hypothesis. Our case study gives us evidence, at the 5% significance level, to conclude that smoking is likely to be associated with chest disease.

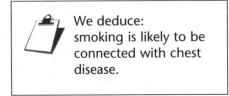

We deduce: smoking is likely to be connected with chest disease.

For our second case study (investigating whether H.E.G. support makes a significant contribution to success in quitting smoking) we have '2' degrees of freedom, and calculated χ^2 = 8.58. Here we see that '8.58' is greater than the value 'χ = 5.99' which the Table tells us is the

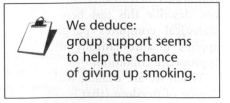

We deduce: group support seems to help the chance of giving up smoking.

boundary of the 5% critical region. Thus our value lies in the critical region, which justifies us in discarding the null hypothesis. So at the 5% significance level we reject the null hypothesis and we accept that it is likely that the Health Education Group makes a significant difference to people giving up smoking.

Suppose we wish to test the null hypothesis in our second case study at a higher level of significance, namely at the 1% significance level. From the Table (Appendix 5(d)), when there are two degrees of freedom the critical region at the 1% significance level is bounded by the value '$\chi^2 = 9.21$'. Since our calculated value is '$\chi^2 = 8.58$' which is *less than* '9.21', this result is *not* in the critical region. Thus at the 1% significance level we do not have enough evidence to reject the null hypothesis; from the results of this particular sample – at this (more rigorous) level of significance.

11.4 Improving the result from a χ^2 test

Although the χ^2 test is usually applied using a computer package, we have indicated above the basic way it works. To be sure that it gives us a valid result, however, there are some warnings to be heeded.

The overall frequency should be no less than '50'; in practice we can easily ensure that we do not apply the test to a group of fewer than fifty people.

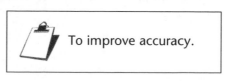
Warning!

No cell should contain an expected frequency of less than '5'. The risk of a cell containing a very small expected value, or even zero, is greatly increased when we deal with **large contingency tables**, those that are '5 × 5' or bigger. To counteract this problem it is sometimes possible to 'combine cells', that is to reduce the number of categories for one of the variables, to ensure that all expected frequencies are '5' or more. Another approach – with contingency tables larger than '2 × 2' – is to 'proceed with caution', so long as *none* of the cells have expected frequencies of less than '1', and *no more than a fifth* of the cells have expected frequencies less than '5'. If we cannot meet these last conditions then an alternative test called **Fisher's exact test** can be used; we will not describe this test here, but the statistical computer package SPSS applies it automatically under the appropriate conditions.

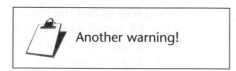
Another warning!

When we are dealing with just '1' degree of freedom (that is, all '2 × 2'

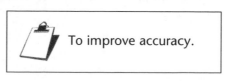
To improve accuracy.

contingency tables) then the accuracy of the result is improved if we apply **Yates' correction**. This involves subtracting ½ from each value of 'O – E' (or 'E – O', whichever of these is a *positive* number) *before* squaring it. Applying Yates' correction, the calculation done for each cell is:

$$\frac{[(O–E) – ½]^2}{E} \text{ if (O – E) is positive}$$

$$\text{or } \frac{[(E–O) – ½]^2}{E} \text{ if (E – O) is positive}$$

These numbers are then added, as before, to get the value of X^2 for the table.

We illustrate the effect of Yates' correction on the figures in our first case study (Section 11.1). Using Tables 11.2 and 11.3, the calculation of χ^2 becomes:

$$\chi^2 = \frac{[(31 – 25) – ½]^2}{25} + \frac{[(31 – 25) – ½]^2}{25} + \frac{[(31 – 25) – ½]^2}{25}$$

$$+ \frac{[(31 – 25) – ½]^2}{25}$$

$$\chi^2 = \frac{(6 – ½)^2}{25} + \frac{(6 – ½)^2}{25} + \frac{(6 – ½)^2}{25} + \frac{(6 – ½)^2}{25}$$

$$= \frac{5.5^2}{25} + \frac{5.5^2}{25} + \frac{5.5^2}{25} + \frac{5.5^2}{25}$$

$$= 1.21 + 1.21 + 1.21 + 1.21$$

$$= 4.84$$

From the Table for χ^2 (Appendix 5(d)), with '1' degree of freedom we know that the critical region for 5% significance is bounded by the value '$\chi^2 = 3.84$'. Now that we have applied Yates' correction, our figure of '4.84' is *still* greater than '3.84' so it is *still* in the critical region; it remains true that our figures give us reason to discard the null hypothesis. Applying this more accurate test we again reach the conclusion we reached earlier: at the 5% significance level we conclude that smoking *is* probably associated with chest disease.

SPSS automatically applies Yates' correction to all χ^2 tests on '2 × 2' contingency tables.

The Strength of Relationships

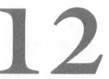

– using scatter diagrams, correlation and regression to quantify relationships between variables

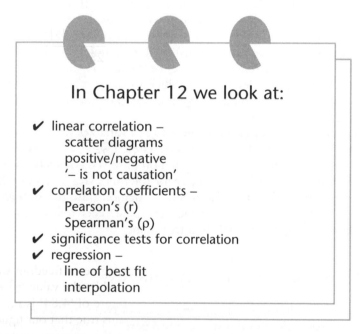

In Chapter 12 we look at:

✔ linear correlation –
    scatter diagrams
    positive/negative
    '– is not causation'
✔ correlation coefficients –
    Pearson's (r)
    Spearman's (ρ)
✔ significance tests for correlation
✔ regression –
    line of best fit
    interpolation

People often suppose on the basis of 'common sense' that certain phenomena are *connected:* this occurs in areas of health, as well as in other aspects of life. We may believe that there is a connection between the number of hours we sleep in a night and the extent to which we feel 'rested' the next day; between the dose of analgesic given to a patient and (within limits) the extent of the pain relief; or between the amount of rehabilitation a person receives and the success of that rehabilitation.

In Chapter 11 we discussed how we can investigate whether such effects are independent – totally unrelated – or not; the results we obtained were either 'they are probably independent' or 'they are probably not independent'. In this chapter we look at ways to *measure the strength* of any such possible connections – graphically and by calculation, using both parametric and non-parametric tests. We also look at when and how we can link variables precisely so that we can predict the value of one effect when we are given an associated value.

12.1 What correlation is

The 'common sense' examples mentioned above can be quite persuasive. However, we must beware of claiming that a connection between effects exists when, in reality, there is none at all; it is sometimes too easy to give in to wishful thinking. When two effects *are* related, then we say that there is a **correlation** between the variables describing these effects. If we can establish a correlation between variables then we can sometimes draw conclusions about the corresponding effects. For instance if we can demonstrate a correlation between 'clinical depression' and 'propensity to succumb to a viral illness', then we can say that the more serious the level of depression suffered by a patient, the more likely they are to develop a viral illness (and also vice versa – the more likely someone is to succumbing to a viral illness then the more likely they are to be suffering from clinical depression).

By calculating a **level of correlation** between variables we can *quantify* the strength of the connection between effects. These figures allow us to compare relationships and so to justify changes based on observed connections. The case for administering additional analgesic, or for offering extra hours of rehabilitation, is more likely to be successful when we demonstrate the *strength* of the correlations, that is, the *extent* to which the pain relief follows the drug or the rehabilitation follows the increased treatment.

12.2 Showing correlation graphically

A very easy way to illustrate whether the values of two variables are connected is via a **scatter diagram**. For this we have two perpendicular axes meeting at the origin (as in a 'standard' graph): the values of one variable are given using the scale on one axis, the values of the second variable using the scale on the other axis (the variables must be measured at interval or ratio level). We here look at scatter diagrams which illustrate the simplest form of correlation, called **linear correlation**, where the points tend to gather along the direction of a straight line.

We consider an example where we are checking for a possible connection between the quantity (A) of an iron-rich drug administered to a patient, and the subsequent haemoglobin count (B) in their blood. The variable (A), 'quantity of drug administered', is measured along the horizontal x-axis and the variable (B), 'haemoglobin count', is measured along the vertical y-axis

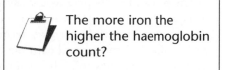

The more iron the higher the haemoglobin count?

(both variables here are measured at ratio level). From a succession of clinical trials we obtain sets of paired figures: when (A) takes value 'a', then (B) takes value 'b'. For each value 'a' there is a corresponding value 'b', and for each pair of these values we plot on our graph the point with co-ordinates (a, b) (see Figure 12.1(i)). Each clinical result gives us another point on the graph – these points may end up appearing like a cloud of points scattered across the page.

Maybe the points we get from our results look like Figure 12.1(i), where they seem to be scattered randomly across the graph without any apparent pattern. This shows us no particular relationship between the variables in this case; we can see no connection at all between the quantity of the drug administered and the patients' haemoglobin counts.

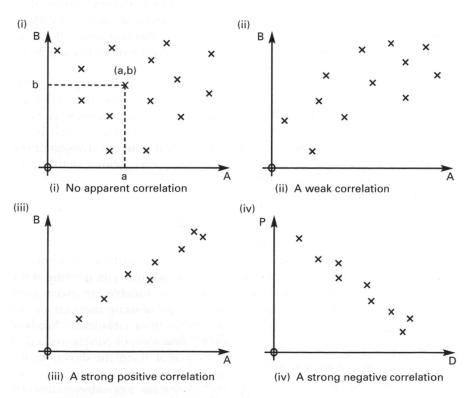

Figure 12.1 Arrangements of points in scatter diagrams

Perhaps our results give us a diagram like that in Figure 12.1(ii), where the points are not randomly scattered but seem to show an overall spread from 'bottom left to top right'. This is termed **positive correlation**: we see that the *smaller* values 'a' correspond with the *smaller* values 'b' and the *larger* values 'a' with the *larger* values 'b'. This diagram shows a **weak correlation**; we infer a general tendency for the haemoglobin count to rise with the increased quantity of the drug administered.

Most likely our results give us a diagram like that of Figure 12.1(iii); here the scatter of points lies very clearly along the direction of a line 'bottom left to top right'. Again this is a positive correlation, but this is a **strong correlation** between the variables, which suggests that the quantity of the drug given is definitely connected to the haemoglobin count.

Figure 12.1(iv) shows a scatter graph which might arise when we are testing for a connection between the variable (D) 'the post-operative dose of analgesic given to a patient' and the variable (P)

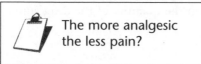
The more analgesic the less pain?

'the amount of pain experienced by a patient after a surgical procedure'. In this case the points are spread along the line from 'top left to bottom right', with the *smaller* values of (D) corresponding with the *larger* values of (P) and vice versa; this is a **negative correlation**. This suggests, as we would expect, that smaller doses of analgesic are associated with higher experience of pain and larger doses of analgesic are associated with lower experience of pain.

12.3 Correlation is not causation

When two effects are related it is all too easy to assume that one of them *must cause* the other. Admittedly it is plausibly true that causality is involved in the above examples: the iron-rich drug probably does increase the haemoglobin count and the analgesic probably does lead to the pain relief. However, it is very misleading to conclude that such relationships are *always* causal. Without

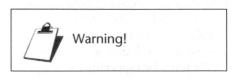
Warning!

firm evidence to the contrary (about the known and intended effects of drugs, for example) we should always believe that *Correlation does not mean causation*.

Here is a simple example to remind us that just because effects are connected we cannot assume that one causes the

Warning: passing urine does not cause fatigue!

other. Suppose we take a survey of women at different times during the progress of their pregnancies, and record particularly their reported levels of tiredness (variable (T)), and the frequency they experience in passing urine (variable (F)). From each woman at each time we obtain a pair of figures: 't' is the value of (T), her tiredness level, and 'f' is the value of (F), the frequency she is experiencing. We use all the pairs of 't' and 'f' to plot points with co-ordinates (t, f) on a scatter diagram. We know that, in general terms, levels of fatigue increase during pregnancy and also the frequency of passing urine increases during pregnancy. As a result, it is *very likely* that our scatter graph demonstrates *positive correlation* between the variables. However, we do *not* deduce that 'tiredness causes women to pass urine more frequently', *nor* do we deduce that 'frequency in passing urine causes tiredness'! Each of the effects *separately* is a consequence of the woman being pregnant. Correlation is *not* the same as causation.

Other examples are less clear-cut, and we must take great care over interpreting the results. Suppose we are interested in finding whether there is any connection between a 'talk therapy', such as counselling, and the psychological well-being of a 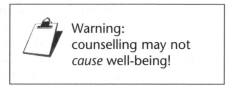 Warning: counselling may not *cause* well-being! patient. We obtain data from a large sample of patients and in each instance we record figures for 'level of psychological well-being' and also 'frequency of counselling sessions' (or 'duration of counselling sessions' or 'number of counselling sessions'). Using the pairs of figures as co-ordinates, we plot points on a scatter diagram: the result may well indicate positive correlation. But will this justify us in concluding that increased counselling *of itself* causes increased psychological well-being? Can we legitimately conclude that 'counselling works' and 'more counselling works better'? Usually it is *not safe* to do so; there may well be other influences at work. For example, the improvement in the reported well-being of the patients may be due to the natural passage of time after a trauma, or it may be due to the extra attention they are receiving (more time for discussions or more frequent visits to look forward to) rather than to the additional counselling as such. The relationship between the counselling and the psychological state may well be spurious: correlation and causation are *different*.

We must be especially careful of drawing conclusions about causation when any relationship between the variables is likely to be controversial. A prime example of this is the possible connection between social class and intellectual development. It is generally accepted (although there are many honourable individual exceptions) that a positive correlation can be demonstrated between social class and intellectual development. However, we make the measurements, in general terms the 'higher' the social class of a

Warning: high social class does not cause a high IQ!

person, then the 'higher' their intellectual development – given by their educational performance. Social scientists may debate both sides of this matter but clearly it is not right for us to conclude that either effect is *caused* by the other: belonging to the upper class does not cause a person to show high intellectual development and performing well educationally does not cause someone to rise in society. Of course we can identify various possible influences. Belonging to the upper class *may* imply having more wealth, which *may* imply greater access to good schools and to books, which *may* imply a greater likelihood of intellectual development. Showing low attainment levels at school *may* confine a person to lowly paid jobs which *may* reduce their apparent social class. But maybe none of these influences applies! – correlation does *not* mean causation.

Despite this serious warning, it can be very worthwhile to identify a correlation. If we have reason to suspect a connection between effects (possibly based on previous biological or pharmacological results) then demonstrating correlation between the variables is a valuable exercise. The existence of correlation can also encourage us to speculate on causation and to devise methods to test for that; correlation can often point us towards promising avenues of investigation. We would be unjustified, however, in gathering large amounts of disparate data and embarking on a 'fishing trip' for relationships based on correlation between variables – without any theoretical basis.

12.4   Calculating the level of correlation

A figure which represents the *strength* of the relationship between variables is called a **level of correlation**. So far, in identifying a correlation and drawing a scatter diagram, we have used paired figures: a sample of values of one variable paired up with a sample of values of another variable (the 'pairs' usually refer to related data samples which arise from one individual, or one time). To find a level of correlation we calculate the **correlation coefficient**, **r**, which depends on *all* the pairs of figures. This coefficient is often called **Pearson's correlation coefficient**, or sometimes the **product moment correlation coefficient**. Here we shall *describe* this calculation; obviously in reality we expect to use a computer package to perform it for us.

Suppose the two variables we are dealing with are X and Y. We have n values of X (we call each of these 'x'), and they correspond to n values of Y, each called 'y'. Altogether our scatter diagram shows n points, labelled by the co-ordinates (x, y).

We take the sample of all the 'x s', and calculate the sample mean $\bar{x}$ and the sample standard deviation s_x (see Sections 5.2 and 5.3). Similarly, from the sample of all the 'y s' we calculate the sample mean $\bar{y}$ and the sample standard deviation s_y.

Now for each pair of x and y we calculate what look rather similar to z-scores. In fact we calculate:

$$\frac{x - \bar{x}}{s_x} \quad \text{and} \quad \frac{y - \bar{y}}{s_y}$$

These are *not* the z-scores that we met in Section 6.4 because the number under each fraction here is the *sample* standard deviation (not σ the *population* standard deviation). For each pair of x and y we multiply the above fractions to get their 'product':

$$\frac{x - \bar{x}}{s_x} \times \frac{y - \bar{y}}{s_y}$$

We obtain the correlation coefficient by adding all these products together (for all the pairs of figures we have) then dividing the total by 'n', which is the number of pairs. The correlation coefficient, the r-score, is:

$$r = \frac{1}{n} \sum \left(\frac{x - \bar{x}}{\sigma_x} \times \frac{y - \bar{y}}{\sigma_y} \right)$$

The r-score is always a number between '−1' and '+1'. The *size* of 'r' indicates the strength of the relationship between the variables: the closer the size is to '1', then the stronger the relationship. As a rule of thumb, correlations where the size of the r-score is 0.3 or less are considered weak correlations and correlations where the size of the r-score is over 0.7 are considered strong correlations. The *sign (plus or minus)* of 'r' tells us the 'direction' of the relationship: if 'r' is positive there is positive correlation between the variables and if 'r' is negative there is negative correlation.

When 'r' is close to zero then clearly no (linear) correlation has been detected. What can we deduce from this? Maybe there really is no correlation present at all. On the other hand, there might be a correlation that our method has not picked up. This could have happened if we had truncated the scales before we calculated the r-score for a restricted number of pairs of values. Such a truncation could mask the presence even of a strong correlation such as that shown in the scatter diagram of Figure 12.2. Another possibility is that a curvilinear correlation exists, which a scatter diagram might suggest but our calculation for linear correlation would not identify. We illustrate a **curvilinear correlation** in Figure 12.3: there is an obvious connection between the ages of boys and men and their hand grip strength, but the points follow the direction of a curve rather than a single straight line so the r-score is close to zero. These examples show how useful scatter diagrams can be in indicating possible correlations; we should not rely solely on calculations.

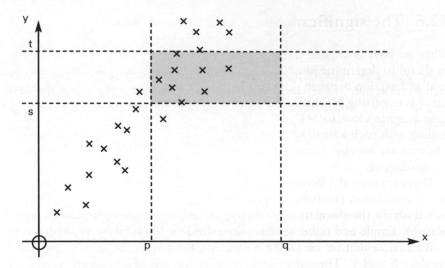

There is obviously an overall strong correlation between values of x and values of y. But the points in the truncated part of the diagram shaded show zero correlation.

Figure 12.2 Truncation can mask correlation

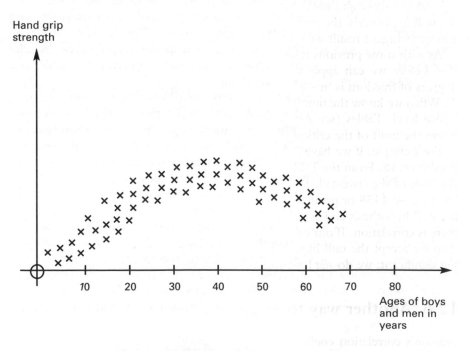

Figure 12.3 A curvilinear correlation

12.5 The significance of a correlation level

When we have calculated the correlation coefficient for a pair of variables it can be useful to determine just how *significant* the correlation is: does it indicate a 'real' connection between the variables? or is it possible that the apparent correlation is occurring by chance? It may be, for instance, that although the coefficient is quite close to '+1', the result is not really significant because we are dealing with such a small sample. Especially when we get an r-score which is an intermediate number (such as 0.5, say) it is valuable to have a way of assessing its significance.

There are several different methods which can be used to test the significance of the correlation coefficient, the r-score. One of them uses *t*-scores, another uses 'Fisher's transformation' and then z-scores. The one we mention here is relatively simple and rather similar to the chi-squared test.

We assume that we are working with random samples of values taken by the variables X and Y. The correlation coefficient, the r-score that we have calculated, is a single *sampling statistic*. Our null hypothesis is that the corresponding *population parameter* – the correlation coefficient for the whole population – is zero, so that there is no correlation at all. Applying a 5% significance test, we see whether the calculated r-score lies among the extreme 5% of all possible values. If the r-score *does* lie among the extreme 5% of all values then we reject the null hypothesis and say that 'r' *is* significant and correlation *is* likely. If the calculated r-score *does not* lie among the extreme 5% of all values then we accept the null hypothesis: the result *is not* significant, and correlation is unlikely. For a more stringent result we can apply a 1% significance test.

As with some previous tests, we need to know the number of *degrees of freedom* before we can apply this significance test. For this test the number of degrees of freedom is '$n - 2$', that is, 'the number of pairs of observations, less 2'. When we know the number of degrees of freedom, and have agreed a significance level, Tables (see Appendix 5e) tell us the value of the r-score which marks the limit of the critical region.

For example, if we have 20 pairs of observations, the number of degrees of freedom is 18. From the Table in Appendix 5(e) we read that '$r = 0.4438$' marks the limit of the (two-tailed) 5% critical region. Thus if our calculated r-score is less than -0.4438 or greater than $+0.4438$, it is in the critical region: we reject the null hypothesis and state that it *is* significantly likely (at the 5% level) that there is correlation. If our calculated r-score lies between -0.4438 and $+0.4438$ then we accept the null hypothesis and state that (at the 5% level) our result is *not* significant; we do *not* have sufficient evidence to say there is correlation.

12.6 Another way to calculate a level of correlation

Pearson's correlation coefficient, described above, is a *parametric* measure of correlation where – implicitly – we assume that the variables under consideration are measured at interval or ratio level and are normally distributed. There is also a well known *non-parametric* measure of correlation called **Spearman's rank-correlation coefficient**, which uses the **symbol ρ** (the Greek letter 'r', pronounced like the 'ro' in 'rose'). This allows us to quantify any correlation between samples of observations without needing information about the populations from which they come; it is especially useful when the variables are measured at an ordinal level only.

> Does a student prioritise like an experienced clinician?

An example where it is appropriate to calculate Spearman's rank-correlation coefficient is when a student (S) is given the task of prioritising, on the basis of their own clinical judgement, the treatment of a group of ten patients. The ordering they give is compared with that of an experienced clinician (L); just how different are the two orderings?

The outcome of this exercise is shown in Table 12.1. The ten patients are indicated by the letters A to J. Table 12.1(a) shows the *ranked* (that is, ordered) list drawn up by the student (S); Table 12.1(b) shows the corresponding ranked list drawn up by the experienced clinician (L). In Table 12.1(c) these lists are combined, and against the 'name' of each patient we see the two rankings, one due to (S) and the other due to (L).

It is easy to calculate the rank-correlation coefficient, the ρ-score. From Table 12.1(c), looking at each patient in turn we find the *difference* in the two rankings. Thus if patient A is ranked 'S_A' by the student, and 'L_A' by the experienced clinician, we calculate:

Table 12.1 The ordering of patients, priorities allocated by the student (S) and by the experienced clinician (L)

(a) Priority allocated by (S)

Ranking:	1st	2nd	3rd	4th	5th	6th	7th	8th	9th	10th
Patient:	B	G	C	J	A	F	D	I	E	H

(b) Priority allocated by (L)

Ranking:	1st	2nd	3rd	4th	5th	6th	7th	8th	9th	10th
Patient:	C	J	G	B	F	A	E	I	D	H

(c) Comparison of the two rankings

Patient:	A	B	C	D	E	F	G	H	I	J
Ranking (S)	5	1	3	7	9	6	2	10	8	4
Ranking (L)	6	4	1	9	7	5	3	10	8	2

$S_A - L_A$

and we square this, giving:

$(S_A - L_A)^2$

We do this for each patient in turn and add up the total:

$\sum (S - L)^2$

From this (where n is the number of patients) we calculate Spearman's rank-correlation coefficient:

$$\rho = 1 - \frac{6 \times \sum (S - L)^2}{n(n^2 - 1)}$$

In our example we have (adding for the ten patients):

$$
\begin{aligned}
\sum (S - L)^2 &= (5 - 6)^2 + (1 - 4)^2 + (3 - 1)^2 + (7 - 9)^2 + (9 - 7)^2 \\
&\quad + (6 - 5)^2 + (2 - 3)^2 + (10 - 10)^2 + (8 - 8)^2 \\
&\quad + (4 - 2)^2 \\
&= 1 + 9 + 4 + 4 + 4 + 1 + 1 + 0 + 0 + 4 = 28
\end{aligned}
$$

Putting this into the formula for ρ (with n = 10) we get:

$$\rho = 1 - \frac{6 \times 28}{10 \times 99} = 1 - \frac{168}{999} = 1 - 0.170 = 0.83$$

(working to 2 decimal place accuracy).

Just the same as Pearson's correlation coefficient, the Spearman's rank-correlation coefficient takes values between '−1' and '+1' to indicate the *strength* of the correlation between variables. When 'ρ = +1' we have complete positive correlation between the variables (that is, the two orders match exactly); when 'ρ = −1' we have complete negative correlation between the variables (that is, the two rankings are in precisely opposite order). When 'ρ' is close to zero, then there is very little correlation at all. Thus for our example above, where Spearman's rank-correlation coefficient is 0.83, we have a fairly strong positive correlation between the ranking given by the student and that given by the experienced clinician: there is a fairly high level of agreement between their prioritisation.

As we have seen, it is straightforward to calculate 'ρ' to compare corresponding rankings in any two, fairly short, lists. The ranking can be assigned *qualitatively*, as above, or it may be due to *quantitative* differences; it can be

Table 12.2   Dealing with a tie in rankings

Original ranked order of categories: F, E, (B, C), A, D

Table of rankings:

Categories	A	B	C	D	E	F
Assigned ranking	5	3½	3½	6	2	1

presented in ascending or descending order. Caution is needed if there are *many* 'ties' in the two rankings, but, in practice, if we are given just a few 'ties' the method needs only slight modification. Suppose we have the order

F, E, (B, C), A, D

where B and C are tied as 'joint third' out of the six categories. In this case the ranking number given to both is '3½' (the average of the '3' and '4' of their order as written). Table 12.2 shows these rankings.

We can also use our calculation of 'Spearman's ρ' to determine whether the correlation is statistically significant (at the 5% level, say). The null hypothesis is that the correlation is *not* significant and any apparent matching of the two rankings occurs merely by chance. The table in Appendix 5(f) uses 'n' (the number of categories) to give us the value of 'ρ' that marks the boundary of the critical region, at 5% or 1% significance levels. If our calculated ρ-score is *larger* than the value in the table (for a one-tailed test) or *numerically larger, ignoring the + or − sign* (for a two-tailed test) then we know that our result is significant. In our example above n = 10, and the table in Appendix 5(f) gives the value '$\rho = 0.648$' as the boundary of the critical region for a two-tailed test at 5% significance in this case. Thus our calculated value, $\rho = 0.83$, indicates a significant result. We reject the null hypothesis because our value is in the critical region and we deduce that we probably have a real correlation here, one that is unlikely to have come about just by chance.

12.7 Regression

As we have been discussing in the above sections, correlation is essentially descriptive. It allows us to identify *how strong* a relationship is between variables, the *direction* of that relationship, and whether it is *likely* that any such relationship occurs other than by mere chance. The first two of these features are illustrated in Figure 12.4 where we see that the points in the scatter diagram are fairly well aligned in a positive direction (bottom left to top right) so we deduce that there is a fairly strong correlation between the variables X and Y. However, correlation does *not* allow us to deduce where additional points on a scatter diagram might lie and it does *not* give us any tools to work out a precise relationship between variables.

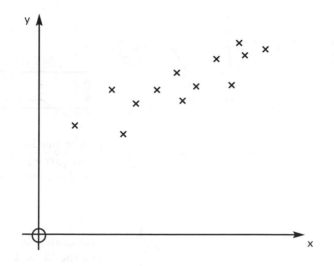

Figure 12.4   A scatter diagram showing positive correlation

So what might we do if we have some correlated data and we wish to infer the value of one variable from a known value of the other variable? As an example, suppose we have a positive correlation between a sample of 'hours spent in a hospital bed' by a group of patients and 'quantity of pressure sores developed'. For any particular figure for the 'hours spent in bed' offered, we might wish to deduce the expected 'quantity of pressure sores developed' (without performing the experiment!). Or we might identify a particular 'quantity of pressure sores developed' and wish to find the corresponding figure for the 'hours spent in bed'. The tool we use in these cases is called **regression**.

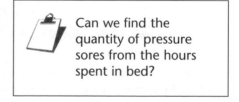

Can we find the quantity of pressure sores from the hours spent in bed?

Where we are sure that we do have correlation between two variables (measured at interval or ratio level), regression allows us to identify a precise relationship between them and also to interpolate, that is, to 'fill the gaps' between points on the scatter diagram. Here we are dealing with **(simple) linear regression**, so we apply methods of regression to find the **line of best fit** in a scatter diagram. This gives us a *formula* for the precise relationship between the variables. If we are given a value of one variable, the formula allows us to *calculate* the corresponding value of the other – in other words we are able to *predict* values.

On a 'standard' graph the horizontal axis is the **x-axis** and the vertical axis is the **y-axis**; they meet at the **origin**, where both their **scales** show zero. The

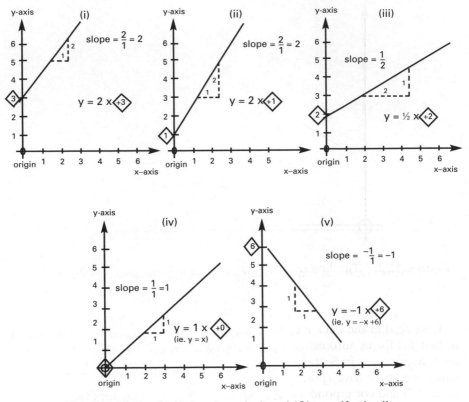

Figure 12.5 Showing how 'm' and 'C' specify the line

essential features of a straight line on a standard graph are its **slope** or **gradient** and its **y-intercept** – the point where it cuts the y-axis. When we know its slope (referred to as 'm') and its y-intercept (say at the point where y = C) we immediately have enough information to specify the line (see Figures 12.5(i),(ii),(iii),(iv),(v)). The 'name' of a straight line on a graph is the formula:

y = mx + C

where 'm' and 'C' are the actual numbers for the gradient and the y-intercept. (This is sometimes called '*the equation of the straight line*'.) When we know a particular value 'x', we can put it into the formula and calculate the corresponding value 'y' (and vice versa).

The technique of regression allows us to use the paired values of variables to calculate figures for 'm' and 'C' and so draw the line of best fit onto a scatter diagram. In Figure 12.6 we show the line of best fit superimposed on the points in the scatter diagram of Figure 12.4. The method for calculating the line of best fit is also called the **method of least squares**, as its theory deals with minimising the total of the 'squares' of all the vertical distances shown in the diagram.

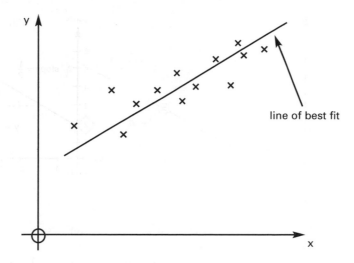

Figure 12.6 The line of best fit for the points of Figure 12.4 (showing the vertical distances)

If we feed in the data, a computer package calculates a regression line (line of best fit) for us automatically; here we just describe the type of calculations used. Suppose, as in Section 12.4, we are dealing with two variables X and Y which we know have (positive) correlation. We have 'n' values of X (each is called 'x') and corresponding to each of these we have a value of Y, called 'y'. Our scatter diagram contains n points, with co-ordinates (x, y).

To find the line of best fit through these points, we first calculate the mean of all the 'xs' (call this x̄) and the mean of all the 'ys' (call this ȳ). The line of best fit passes through the point (x̄, ȳ), which we can think of as a *pivot point* on the line and mark on the graph (see Figure 12.7).

Next we calculate the slope of the line. From each value of 'x' we subtract the mean, x̄, and then multiply what is left by the corresponding 'y' value. We add up the total of these n results, giving:

$$\sum [(x - \bar{x}) \times y]$$

Dividing this by the total of the 'squares' of all the (x − x̄) terms gives the slope:

$$m = \frac{\sum [(x - \bar{x}) \times y]}{\sum (x - \bar{x})^2}$$

Since the pivot point lies on the line, and we now know the numerical value of the slope 'm', we calculate the value of 'C' (the y-intercept) from the equation:

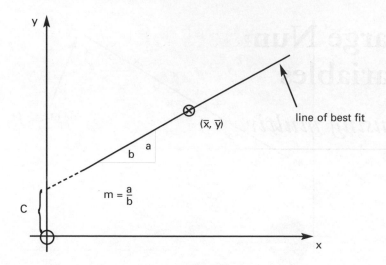

Figure 12.7   The line of best fit, showing the pivot point and indicating 'm' and 'C'

$$\bar{y} = m\,\bar{x} + C$$

Now we know 'm' and 'C', so we have the formula for the line of best fit:

$$y = m\,x + C$$

We can use this line of best fit to predict (as yet unknown) values of the variables. For instance, if we are interested in a particular value (say $x = x_0$) of the variable X, we can put that number into the above formula of the straight line and calculate the associated (predicted) value, y_0, of the variable Y. The value is given by:

$$y_0 = m\,x_0 + C$$

Here we have actually found and used the **regression line of Y on X**, as in the working we have assumed that the values of 'x' are the ones we know about and the values of 'y' are the ones we might wish to calculate/predict. If we were to do the calculations to obtain the **regression line for X on Y** we would obtain a slightly different value for 'm', but for many purposes this is not important.

Large Numbers of Variables

13

– *using multivariate methods of analysis*

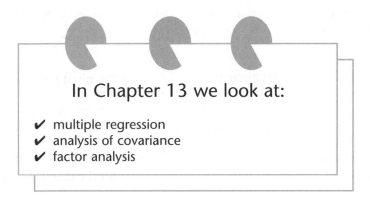

In Chapter 13 we look at:

✔ multiple regression
✔ analysis of covariance
✔ factor analysis

All of us will agree that *real* life is seldom simple – in fact it is usually very complicated! The statistical tools we have discussed so far are only useful if we can isolate the particular features in which we are interested (preferably looking at them one or two at a time); but in practice we are very likely to wish to make sense of *large* datasets, where it may not be clear how we should disentangle information about different features. We have an example of one such large data set in Chapter 2, where from the questionnaire of Table 2.3 we obtained the data in Table 2.5: in the subsequent sections we did not attempt to analyse that *as a whole*, instead we focused on individual variables, one by one.

Another large dataset could come from a fairly standard patient survey, which includes demographic data such as age, gender, home post-code, diagnosis and clinical area, as well as answers filled in by each patient regarding their admission and stay in hospital, their satisfaction with different aspects of their care and their feelings about their physical and psychological well-being. If we wish to find the relative effects of all the variables concerned here, and to discover which of the demographic variables, say, is most important in influencing the other answers, then we could deal with the variables singly or in pairs – a laborious process! But it would be more efficient to apply **multivariate**

methods of analysis. These techniques, some of which we outline below, allow us to look at the relationships between a large number of variables *in one step*, and to investigate the effects of different variables *in the presence of other variables*.

It is beyond the scope of this book to deal with multivariate methods in any detail. In this final chapter we indicate what can be achieved using some multivariate methods; we sketch out general principles of how the techniques work and show that they are based on familiar ideas that we have introduced in earlier chapters.

As with all the other statistical methods we have met, multivariate methods can be performed using a statistical computer package. When we have *many* variables, 'pen and calculator' methods of analysis involve heroic quantities of arithmetic; multivariate methods involve quite complex procedures so we do not expect to do these calculations ourselves.

13.1 Multiple regression

In Section 12.7 we looked at the simplest form of regression, *simple linear regression*. By identifying the *line of best fit* we found a precise relationship between a pair of variables, and could then deduce unknown values of one of them by *interpolation*. For the *regression of Y on X* we have the formula for the line of best fit:

$$y = m x + C$$

Here we assume that the values 'x', which are values of the variable X, are the ones we know about, and that these then determine the corresponding values 'y' of the variable Y: the 'y' values depend on the 'x' values. We are assuming that the variable X is influencing the variable Y as, for example,

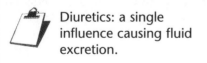
Diuretics: a single influence causing fluid excretion.

we would generally assume that the quantity of a diuretic administered determines the quantity of fluid excreted – and not vice versa. In such a case we call X the **independent variable** and Y is the **dependent variable**.

In the 'real world' it is relatively unusual for there to be a simple relationship between two variables which is totally independent of the influence of any other variable. We more usually have several different independent variables, sometimes called **predictor variables** or **covariates**, which together influence another – dependent – variable. For example we would assume that the

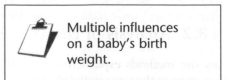
Multiple influences on a baby's birth weight.

birth weight of a baby is influenced by many variables, including the nutrition of the mother, the stature of both the mother and the father, whether the mother smokes and the length of the pregnancy: each of these *independently* affects the birth weight.

We should always be aware of the possibility of multiple influences on any observed effect. For example, regarding the rehabilitation of stroke victims, we can establish relatively easily that the number of hours of physiotherapy given is important and relates to the outcome of rehabilitation. But it surely gives an unreal impression to imply that it is *only* the number of hours of physiotherapy that affects the reconstruction

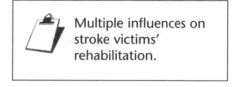

Multiple influences on stroke victims' rehabilitation.

of capabilities leading to an acceptable way of life? What about the age of the patient? Are they male or female? Are they married? How mentally active were they before the stroke? What was their initial level of fitness? Do they enjoy music? Were they overweight to begin with? What level of support do they get from their family? Did they play golf? It is obvious that there are many other variables which *might* influence the rehabilitation.

Multiple regression allows us to compare the influence of more than one independent variable on a dependent variable, at the same time. Thus we can determine which independent variable most 'explains' the changes in the dependent variable, and calculate the extent to which this occurs. This gives us a better understanding of the relative influences in a situation. To analyse a case using multiple regression we look at the regression of one dependent variable, Y, on several independent variables, say X_1, X_2, X_3, X_4, and X_5; the regression formula looks like this:

$$y = m_1x_1 + m_2x_2 + m_3x_3 + m_4x_4 + m_5x_5 + C$$

where the 'm s' and 'C' are all numbers. We see that this is similar to the formula for simple regression.

In the example on stroke victims' rehabilitation, it could turn out that certain of the independent variables we proposed have little or no effect on the dependent variable; multiple regression allows us to quantify this, and also to find the statistical significance of any relationships which do exist. It could well be discovered that 'age' has the major effect on the outcome of 'rehabilitation'; this is valuable information. We would then know that a person's age should be taken into account, as well as the number of hours of physiotherapy allocated, when aiming for a given level of rehabilitation.

13.2 Analysis of covariance

By the methods explained in Section 9.4 we can test whether 'large' samples come from the same population. When we have *estimated* the standard deviation of the population in question we use a t-score (in an independent t-test) to test whether the two samples are both likely to have come from that population. However, for this test to give us an unequivocally significant result we must assume that the two samples are well chosen, and unbiased with respect to the variables we are comparing. There are cases when they might not be, and there might be an in-built bias – as we illustrate in the following example.

Suppose that we have two large samples, one of men and one of women. We wish to test the hypothesis that there is no significant difference between them with regard to their 'social isola-

> Influences on social
> isolation.

tion', that is they (probably) come from the same population. We might assume that we are dealing only with the variables 'gender' and 'social isolation' here, and by the independent t-test we might indeed find that there is a significant difference between the samples (so they probably do *not* come from the same population). But on closer inspection we may see that another variable is involved: the average age of the men is ten years more than the average age of the women – might this be having some effect on the result?

To test whether this third variable has a significant effect we carry out an **analysis of covariance** which takes into account the influences of both gender and age on each group. If the result remains statistically significant then 'age' *did not* affect the outcome, but if the result is no longer statistically significant then 'age' *did* affect the outcome.

A variable like 'age', as in this case, can be an unforeseen cause of bias in an investigation; it can either amplify or else mask the effect of the variable in which we are principally interested. It is often termed a **confounding variable** and analysis of covariance is the way used to investigate and interpret its effect.

13.3 Factor analysis

There are many occasions when, for convenience, we might wish to group a large number of variables into a smaller number of underlying **factors** or **dimensions**. For example, in a set of patients' records we might wish to record their address, phone number, GP's details, occupation and how many in their household; their gender, height, weight and blood group; their blood

>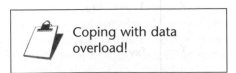
> Coping with data
> overload!

pressure, respiratory rate and heart rate. These could be summarised into data concerning three factors or dimensions: the patients' domestic details, their physical characteristics and their physiological measurements.

The above example is too simple! – in setting it up the underlying dimensions were obvious. But there are occasions when we might be 'flooded' by lists of data referring to *very many variables* measured on a large sample of people. It might appear impossible to connect many of these variables 'by eye' or just using common sense, but the tools of **factor analysis** or **principal component analysis** – based on the concept of *correlation* – allow us to reduce a lengthy list of variables to a compact list reflecting the underlying dimensions.

Factor analysis starts with us calculating all the correlations between all the pairs of variables concerned. We can illustrate the method with a small number: suppose we have just three variables X, Y and Z measured on our sample, then we calculate the correlation coefficient 'r' (see Section 12.4) between each pair, X and Y, Y and Z, and Z and X. The correlation coefficient is 'symmetrical' – that is the correlation between X and Y is the same as that between Y and X – so we can write:

$$r_{XY} = r_{YX}, \text{ etc.}$$

Since the correlation of any variable *with itself* is perfect, we know that:

$$r_{XX} = 1, \text{ etc.}$$

We write these results in a '3 × 3' grid called a '3 × 3' **matrix**, shown in Figure 13.1(a).

In this **correlation matrix**, since the entries in the 'top right' section of the matrix are a mirror image of those in the 'bottom left' section, it is usual to omit one half for convenience. We show the simplified version in Figure 13.1(b).

If we have ten variables then we calculate up to one hundred correlations (not all different) and we place the appropriate coefficients in one half of a '10 × 10' correlation matrix. The **lead diagonal** in the matrix (the diagonal 'top left to bottom right') always contain only '1s', since the correlation coefficient of a variable with itself is '1'. Even presented like this we still have too much data to comprehend easily. We can probably see that some entries are close to zero

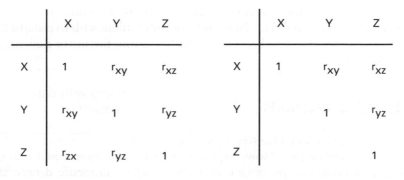

	X	Y	Z			X	Y	Z
X	1	r_{xy}	r_{xz}		X	1	r_{xy}	r_{xz}
Y	r_{xy}	1	r_{yz}		Y		1	r_{yz}
Z	r_{zx}	r_{yz}	1		Z			1

Figure 13.1(a) A '3 × 3' correlation matrix

Figure 13.1(b) The simplified correlation matrix

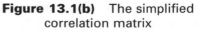

(meaning very weak correlation) and some sets of entries may be close to '1' (meaning very strong correlation) but it is likely that the overall pattern is still far too complex for us to group the variables and to detect factors by eye.

Factor analysis then uses the ideas and techniques of matrix algebra (including **eigenvalues**, **dimensions** and **rotating axes**) to identify, from a correlation matrix, which sets of variables can most appropriately be grouped together into factors; there may be one factor or several. Each of the original variables is assigned a **loading** onto each of the factors: a high loading (generally agreed to be 0.4 or greater) relates the variable to that factor while a low loading means that the variable is not associated with that factor. If there are variables which do not load onto any factor, or **cross load** onto more than one, then conventionally we eliminate these in our search for a **simple structure**.

If we can reduce the data from all the variables to that from a relatively small set of factors then we can be sure that we are obtaining (nearly) all the information in a much more manageable way. The usual aim is to group the variables into as few factors as possible, bearing in mind that each factor should be capable of meaningful interpretation in the scenario considered.

Having obtained a grouping we label the factors, by seeing just how the variables are related. For example, in an analysis of different activities undertaken

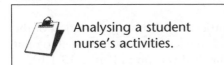

Analysing a student nurse's activities.

by student nurses we might find that the activities 'sitting with a patient' and 'listening to a patient' have high loadings onto the same factor, which we may label 'psychosocial aspects of care', whereas the activities 'measuring vital signs' and 'monitoring for medication side effects' have high loadings onto a different factor, which we can label 'technical aspects of care'. If labelling in this way proves impossible then quite obviously the factor analysis has not produced anything useful: the only remedy is to start again, either by redefining the number of factors required – or by redesigning the questionnaire or experiment!

We have outlined here what is called **exploratory factor analysis**, which allows us to explore data for putative factors. Another technique, known as **confirmatory factor analysis**, allows us to test the validity of a factor structure which may have been guessed at, or reached by exploratory factor analysis; this is not always necessary.

13.4 Other methods

In this and the preceding chapters we have indicated the principal ideas behind basic statistical techniques. However, there are many more methods of statistical analysis in common use in clinical practice and in nursing and healthcare research. We include brief information on some additional statistical methods in the Glossary.

Appendix 1

Further Recommended Reading

(a) Books which include introductions to general statistical concepts and techniques

1. Bryman A, Cramer D (2001)
   Quantitative data analysis with SPSS Release 10 for Windows
   Routledge, London
2. Clarke G M, Cooke D (1978)
   A Basic Course in Statistics
   Edward Arnold, London
3. Harris R L (2000)
   Information Graphics: A comprehensive illustrated reference
   Oxford University Press, Oxford
4. Hayslett M S (1968)
   Statistics made Simple
   W H Allen, London
5. Hinton P R (1995)
   Statistics Explained
   Routledge, London
6. Huff D (1954)
   How to lie with Statistics
   Gollanz, London
7. Owen F, Jones R (1982)
   Statistics
   Pitman, London
8. Spear M E (1952)
   Charting Statistics
   McGraw-Hill, New York
9. Stevens S S (1951)
   Mathematics, Measurement and Psychophysics.
   In Stevens S S (Ed) Handbook of Experimental Psychology, Wiley, NY
10. Stuart A (1984)
    The ideas of sampling
    Griffin, High Wycombe

(b) Books which discuss statistical techniques in the context of nursing and healthcare

1. Altman D G, Machin D, Bryant T N, Gardiner M J (2000)
   Statistics with Confidence (2nd Ed)
   BMJ Books, London
2. Armitage P, Berry G (1987)
   Statistical Methods in Medical Research
   Blackwell, Oxford
3. Bland M, (2000)
   An introduction to medical statistics (3rd Ed)
   OUP, Oxford
4. Coggan D (2003)
   Statistics in Clinical Practice (2nd Ed)
   BMJ Books, London
5. De Vauss D A (1996)
   Surveys in Social Research (4th Ed) (Social Research today; 5)
   UCL Press, London
6. Fowler J, Jarvis P, Chevannes M (2002)
   Practical statistics for nursing and healthcare
   Wiley, London
7. Gardener M J, Altman D G (1986)
   Statistics with Confidence – Confidence Intervals and Statistical Guidelines
   BMJ Books, London
8. Hart A (2001)
   Making sense of statistics in healthcare
   Radcliffe Medical Press, Oxford
9. Moser C A, Kalton G (1985)
   Survey Methods in Social Investigation
   Gower, London
10. Swinslow T D V, Campbell M J (2002)
    Statistics at Square One (10th Ed)
    BMJ Books, London

(c) Papers containing specific research which is referred to in the text

1. Church S, Henderson M, Barnard M, Hart G (2001)
   'Violence by clients towards female prostitutes in different work settings: questionnaire survey'
   British Medical Journal, 322, 524–5
2. Coyle J, Williams B (2001)
   'Valuing people as individuals: development of an instrument through a survey of person-centredness in secondary care'
   Journal of Advanced Nursing, 36(3), 450–9

3. Faugier J, Sargeant M (1997)
   'Sampling hard-to-reach populations'
   Journal of Advanced Nursing, Vol 26, 790–7
4. Mahoney F I, Barthel D W (1965)
   'Functional Evaluation, The Barthel Index'
   Maryland State Medical Journal, 14, 61–5
5. Rhodes T, Donoghoe M, Hunter G, Stimson G V (1994)
   'HIV prevalence no higher among female drug injectors also involved in prostitution'
   AIDS Care, Vol 6, No 3, 269–76
6. Scottish Centre for Infection and Environmental Health (SCIEH) (1995)
   HIV & AIDS Surveillance in Scotland, Review of the Epidemic to December 1994
   SCIEH, Glasgow
7. Shoemaker A L (1996)
   'What's Normal? Temperature, gender and heart rate'
   Journal of Statistics Education, Vol 4, No 2
8. Waterlow J (1985)
   'Pressure sores: a risk assessment card'
   Nursing Times 81(48), 49–55
8. Waterlow J (1991)
   'A policy that protects: the Waterlow pressure sore prevention/treatment policy'
   Professional Nurse, 6(5), 258, 260, 262
9. World Health Organisation (2003)
   International Statistical Classification of Diseases and related Health Problems
   ICD 10th revision

Appendix 2

Those Greek Symbols . . .

It is extremely difficult to describe and develop the basic ideas of statistics without using the symbols which traditionally have been used, which include several letters taken from the Greek alphabet. Because they are often unfamiliar – and somewhat daunting – we include here a full list of the Greek letters that we have used in this book.

Greek letter	How we write it	How we say it	English equivalent	What the letter means in Statistics
α	alpha	'alfa'	a	the level of significance of a test; the probability of a 'type I' error
β	beta	'beeta'	b	the probability of a 'type II' error; the power of a test
μ	mu	'mew'	m	the mean of a population (so we do not confuse it with '$\bar{x}$', the mean of a sample)
ρ	rho	'roe'	r	Spearman's rank-correlation coefficient
σ	sigma	sigma	s	the standard deviation of a population (so we do not confuse it with 's', the standard deviation of a sample)
Σ	sigma	sigma	capital s	'summation' – the instruction to 'add up' all the numbers in a list
χ	chi	'kye'	'ch' as in 'loch'	χ^2 (chi-squared) is a distribution we use to compare proportions obtained from contingency tables

Appendix 3

Glossary

Abscissa: another word for the x-axis, that is the horizontal axis of a graph.

Alpha coefficient: see Cronbach's alpha.

Alternative hypothesis: this expresses that the null hypothesis is false, and it is sometimes called the experimental hypothesis or the hypothesis of difference. If the null hypothesis is rejected then the alternative hypothesis is accepted. The alternative hypothesis is often the prime interest of an investigator.

ANCOVA: see Covariance analysis.

ANOVA: this stands for ANalysis Of VAriance. It is used to test whether three or more samples might come from the same population. The calculations involve obtaining two different estimates for the variance of this population, the 'within-sample' variation and the 'between-sample' variation. The F-test is then applied to the ratio of these estimates.

Approximation: this is the process of estimating a value, or the name given to an estimate close to a true value.

Arithmetic mean: this is the full name of 'the mean'.

Average: this is an informal name for 'the mean'.

Bar chart: a graph used to show the frequencies of nominal and ordinal variables. The frequency of each variable is represented by the height of a bar; the bars are separated by gaps.

Bias: any influence on a study that may distort the results.

Bimodal: a frequency distribution where two separate values or categories have the same maximum frequency.

Binomial distribution: this is the frequency distribution of a discrete variable which counts the number of 'successes' in a given number of trials; each trial has just two possible outcomes, 'success' or 'failure'.

Binomial test: a hypothesis test based on the binomial distribution.

Biserial correlation: a measure of association of two variables collected on each sampling unit where one variable is continuous and the second is binomial, that is, where only two values are possible.

Bonferroni correction: this is applied to reduce the possibility of making a type I error when multiple significance tests are applied. It involves reducing the level of significance at which the null hypothesis could be rejected: the significance level is divided by the overall number of tests.

Categorical: see Nominal.

Cell: a name for a box in a contingency table where a row and a column intersect.

Census: a survey of an entire study population.

Central location: this is a feature of many distributions where the frequencies are observed to cluster around certain 'central' values. These central values, principally the mode, the median and the mean, can be calculated and used to describe the distribution.

Central tendency: see Central location.

Chance: the situation identified when events occur unpredictably, with no perceived pattern or causality.

Chi-squared test: this is mainly used as a test of association between two variables in a contingency table.

Classical approach: this is an approach to probability which involves being able to enumerate all possible outcomes of an event.

Clinical significance: this indicates that the result of a trial is clinically important. Note that even if a study is statistically significant it does not necessarily mean it is clinically significant, that is important in terms of treating patients.

Cluster analysis: a multivariate technique which groups individual items on the basis of their similarities.

Cluster sampling: a sampling method which first identifies all the sampling units as belonging to (equally sized) subsets called clusters, then obtains a sample of the units by selecting a sample of clusters.

Cohen's Kappa: a statistic used to assess the level of agreement between different results when two people ('raters') measure, or rate, categorical (discrete) variables; it is called 'inter-rater reliability'. The value of Kappa ranges from zero to one; by convention 0.7 and above is viewed as a satisfactory level of reliability.

Confidence: the extent to which we can be sure of something, for example the accuracy of an estimate.

Confidence interval: this is a range of values (from low to high) calculated from sample data. The population parameter of interest (often the mean) lies in this interval, with whichever level of confidence, usually 95%, has been chosen.

Confidence limits: the lower and upper end points of a confidence interval.

Confounding variable: a variable that is related to an independent variable and a dependent variable that may make them appear to be related when they are not.

Contingency table: a rectangular array of rows and columns on which can be represented the relationship between two variables.

Continuous variable: this is a variable whose values that can be expressed as whole numbers or fractions (or decimals) or any in-between values – with no 'gaps' possible; for example, height.

Control group: a group of items which do not receive the intervention of interest; they are used in an experiment to provide a baseline against which the effect of an intervention can be measured.

Convenience sample: a sample of units selected solely because they are the most readily available for a study.

Correlation: the effect by which the values of one variable appear to be connected with the values of another.

Correlation coefficient: a number between −1 and +1 which represents the extent to which the values of two variables are associated.

Correlational research: this is statistical research which investigates the relationship between variables.

Covariance: closely related to correlation, this can be calculated as the correlation coefficient between two variables multiplied by the standard deviation of each.

Covariance analysis: this is ANalysis of COVAriance, or ANCOVA, which is used to investigate and interpret the effect of confounding or extraneous variables.

Covariate: one of several different independent variables which together influence another – dependent – variable; comparison of the influences of covariates can be performed by multiple regression. A confounding or extraneous variable that is held constant in covariance analysis to test the relationship between the dependent and independent variables of interest.

Cramer's V: a measure of association between two variables in a contingency table. The V statistic varies between zero and + 1. Below 0.3 signifies a weak association and above 0.6 reflects a strong association.

Critical region: the range of values in a distribution for which, if the study value falls within it, the null hypothesis is rejected.

Cronbach's Alpha: a useful statistic for representing the internal consistency of scores obtained from summated rating scales such as the Likert scale; it is based on the average item correlation in the scale. The value of Cronbach's Alpha lies between 0 and 1, and 0.7 or above is considered satisfactory to support a claim of reasonable internal consistency for scales used in research.

Cumulative bar chart: a type of bar chart which shows the frequencies of variables measured at an ordinal level. The height of the first bar represents the frequency of the first value of the variable. The height of the second bar represents the combined frequencies of the first and second values. The height of the third and subsequent bars similarly indicate the cumulative frequencies.

Cumulative frequency chart: a chart or graph constructed using the values from a cumulative frequency table.

Cumulative frequency curve: a curve which illustrates the cumulative frequencies of a continuous variable.

Cumulative frequency distribution: this is obtained from a frequency distribution by 'accumulating' for each value its own frequency and the frequencies of all the values lower than it.

Cumulative frequency polygon: this is a graph made up of the straight line segments which join the mid-points of the tops of the bars in a cumulative bar chart (for discrete data). For continuous data it consists of straight line segments joining the points made by plotting cumulative frequencies against the upper class boundaries of the grouped data.

Cumulative frequency table: a table containing the values of a variable together with the 'accumulated' frequencies of all the values up to and including each one considered.

Data: a collection of categories, values or facts from which conclusions may be drawn. 'Primary data' are collected specifically for the task in hand; 'secondary data' are gathered from other people's work and/or published materials.

Deciles: the values which occur in an ordered data set at the points which divide the whole range into ten equal portions.

Degrees of freedom: this is the number of independently valued units in a sample. Its value is often required before a significance test (eg t-test, F-test) can be applied.

Dependent variable: a variable whose values are wholly or partially determined by those of another 'independent' variable.

Descriptive statistics: this is the term used for the branch of Statistics involved with organising data by tables and graphs, and also summarising data sets using the measures of central location and dispersion, etc.

Discrete variable: these are qualities or characteristics that can be expressed only in separate categories or separate numbers, for example gender or nationality or numbers of patients.

Dispersion: this describes the extent of the 'spread-out-ness' of data.

Distribution: see Frequency distribution.

Distribution of sample means: the frequency distribution of the set of means of all possible samples taken from a particular population.

Effect size: this is a method of deciding whether identified differences are actually clinically important. It measures the extent of the change brought about in the course of an experiment.

Empirical approach: this is an approach to probability which is based on everyday experience; relative frequencies measured in the past are interpreted as probabilities for the future.

Estimate: to make a judgement as to a value or category without care for absolute precision, or the name given to this value.

F-test: the significance test used in ANOVA.

F-ratio: the ratio (always greater than '1') of the two different estimates for the population variance in ANOVA.

Factor analysis: a multivariate technique for reducing a large number of variables to fewer underlying 'factors' (also called 'dimensions' or 'latent variables').

Fisher's exact test: this test is used for significance testing on 2×2 contingency tables when the conditions for the chi-squared test cannot be met.

Frequency: the number of occurrences of the value of a variable; it answers the question 'How many times?'.

Frequency density: the scale of measurement on the y-axis used for all histograms and frequency distributions of continuous variables.

Frequency distribution: the overall relationship between the values taken by a variable and their frequencies.

Frequency distribution curve: a frequency distribution plotted as a smooth curve on a graph.

Frequency table: a table containing the values of a variable and the frequency of each.

F-score: see F-ratio.

Hazard ratio: this is calculated in survival analysis to summarise the difference between two survival curves. It represents the reduction in the risk of death with treatment compared to that in a control group, over a specified period of time.

Heteroscedascity: this indicates the inequality of the variance of a variable within different sample groups.

Histogram: a graph which represents the frequency distribution of continuous data using rectangles; the areas of the rectangles are proportional to the frequencies of the grouped values.

Homoscedascity: this indicates the equality of the variance of a variable within different sample groups.

Hypothesis: this is an assumption about one or more frequency distributions whose validity can be tested using statistical methods.

Hypothesis testing: the use of statistical methods to test hypotheses.

Ideogram: a symbol used in a pictogram to represent an occurrence of a variable.

Independent events: these are events that are not related, in that the outcome of one has no effect on the outcome of another (for example, two separate tosses of a coin).

Independent variable: a variable whose values are assumed to arise without being influenced by any other variable.

Inferential statistics: this is the term used for the branch of Statistics involved with using sample data to estimate parameters of populations, and for various types of hypothesis testing.

Interpolate: to insert a value between known values by using proportions or another algebraic method.

Inter-quartile range: the range from the first quartile to the third quartile in a frequency distribution or, equivalently, from the 25th percentile to the 75th percentile.

Interval measure: a level of measurement where the categories or values of a variable can be differentiated, they can be meaningfully ranked and the differences between them are assumed to be quantitatively equal.

Kolmogorov-Smirnov one sample test: this assesses the degree to which an observed pattern of categorical frequencies differs from a specified distribution.

Kruskal-Wallis test: a non-parametric test used for comparing more than two sets of ranked data; it is the non-parametric equivalent of ANOVA.

Kurtosis: the extent of 'peakedness' of a distribution curve.

Leptokurtic: this is a description of a frequency distribution curve which has a very pronounced peak with steep sides.

Level of measurement: there are four 'levels' of measurement: nominal, ordinal, interval and ratio; these are applied either according to the nature of the data or, where appropriate, to the requirements of the investigator.

Likert scale: a scale used to measure attitudes. It is based on the responses to a collection of statements representative of a particular attitude, and provides a number which reflects the extent to which a person holds a favourable or unfavourable attitude towards an attitude object.

Line of best fit: the straight line that passes through most points on a scatter diagram, or which minimises its (vertical) distance from all the points. As a result this is the line that best describes the relationship between two variables illustrated on a scatter diagram.

Linear correlation: this is the situation where one variable appears to be dependent on another in such a way that the scatter diagram of the two variables is very close to a straight line.

Linear regression: this involves working out the precise relationship between two variables by fitting a linear equation to sample data. The independent variable generally uses the horizontal scale on a scatter diagram and is termed 'x'. The dependent variable, whose values are to be predicted, uses the vertical axis and is called 'y'.

Logistic regression: this is a non-linear transformation of linear regression used to predict a dependent variable on the basis of independent variables and to determine the percent of variance in the dependent variable which is explained by the independent variables.

Mann-Whitney U test: this is a non-parametric equivalent of the paired t-test. It is used to test whether the difference between two sets of ranked data is statistically significant.

McNemar test: this is a non-parametric test for the significance of changes in before and after experimental designs, i.e. where individuals are used as their own controls and the measurements are either nominal or ordinal. The degree of probability of the value of the test statistic is determined by using the chi-squared distribution.

Mean: this is the most common and most useful measure of central location. A mean of a sample is denoted by '$\bar{x}$', and is calculated by adding together all the values of the variable (measured at interval or ratio level) and then dividing by the total number of them (that is, the total frequency). The mean of a population is denoted by 'μ'.

Measurement: a method of assigning categories or values to observations of a variable.

Median: this is a measure of central location; once a set of data has been placed in ranked order, the median is the middle value.

Mesokurtic: this is a description of a frequency distribution curve which has a 'medium' degree of 'peakedness', approximately the same as a normal curve.

Method of least squares: this is a mathematical method for finding the line of best fit through a set of points by minimising the (squares of) the vertical distances from each point.

Modal class: in a grouped frequency table, this is the class with the greatest frequency.

Mode: this is a measure of central location, it is the most frequently occurring value or category in a distribution.

Multi-modal: a frequency distribution where there is more than one value or category with the same maximum frequency.

Multiple regression: a multivariate technique, using regression, for determining which of a group of independent variables has most influence on a dependent variable.

Multistage sampling: a sampling method using a sequence of different approaches, for example cluster sampling followed by random sampling.

Multivariate: an approach to the analysis of data involving an exploration of the relationships between three or more variables.

Mutually exclusive events: these are events which cannot happen simultaneously.

Negative correlation: a correlation where one variable decreases in value as the other increases.

Negative skew: this is a description of an asymmetrical frequency distribution which has a 'stretched out' tail in the direction of the negative x-axis; its mean is less than its median.

Nominal: this describes values which are differentiated by name only, and not according to a number scale.

Nominal measure: the lowest level of measurement where the categories of the variable can only be differentiated.

Non-parametric test: a statistical test often involving nominal or ordinal measures that makes no assumptions about the parameters of the frequency distributions of the variables.

Normal curve: the symmetrical, bell-shaped curve of the normal distribution.

Normal distribution: this is the most commonly occurring frequency distribution of continuous variables, which arises often in nature.

Null hypothesis: this is the name of the initial assumption in hypothesis testing; it asserts that there is 'no change' from what is known, that things are as expected – it is the 'status quo' position.

Number: a concept of quantity using zero, units and fractions of units.

Numeral: a symbol with which a number is written, for example '3' for the number which is pronounced 'three'.

Odds ratio: this is a way to compare whether the odds of an event occurring is the same for two study groups, eg smokers and non-smokers developing chest disease. The 'odds' for each study group are determined by dividing the number of cases in which the event occurs by the number of cases in which it does not occur. The odds ratio is calculated by the dividing the odds of occurrence for the first group by the odds of occurrence for the second group. If the odds are the same or very similar for each group then the odds ratio is close to 'one'.

Ogive: this word describes the shape of a cumulative frequency curve (it is said to be like one side of an 'ogee arch').

One-tailed test: this is applied in the situation of a hypothesis test where the expectation of possible outcomes is not even handed. The alternative hypothesis is not merely that the null hypothesis is not valid, but rather that an invalid null hypothesis indicates a difference that is anticipated to be in one specified direction. (For example, in a trial of a drug designed to reduce blood pressure the statistical tests can be applied to establish if the experimental group has a significantly *lower* mean blood pressure after treatment than the control group.)

Ordinal measure: a level of measurement where the categories or values of a variable can be differentiated and also ranked.

Ordinate: another word for the y-axis, the vertical axis of a graph.

Origin: the point where the x-axis and the y-axis of a graph intersect, the joint zero on both axes.

Parameter: a quantity such as mean (μ), variance (σ^2) or standard deviation (σ) which characterises a population.

Parametric test: a statistical test in which assumptions are made about the parameters of the frequency distributions of the variables.

Pearson's correlation coefficient (r): this is a parametric measure of correlation.

Percentiles: the values which occur in an ordered data set at the points which divide the whole range into one hundred equal portions.

Pictogram: the use of symbols (called ideograms) to represent frequencies in a diagram.

Pie chart: the representation of the relative frequencies of a set of data by the areas of sectors in a circle.

Platykurtic: this is a description of a frequency distribution curve which has a relatively low, rounded, shallow peak.

Population: the entire set of individuals or items of interest.

Positive correlation: a correlation where one variable increases in value as the other also increases.

Positive skew: this is a description of an asymmetrical frequency distribution which has a 'stretched out' tail in the direction of the positive x-axis; its mean is greater than its median.

Power of a test: this is the probability that a 'correct' decision is made when a hypothesis test is done. It is the probability of rejecting a false null hypothesis (in favour of a specified alternative hypothesis) and can be calculated as 'one minus the probability of a type II error'.

Probability: this is based on the concepts of chance and risk, and refers to the likelihood of an event occurring. When it is expressed numerically 'probability = zero' indicates that an event is impossible, and 'probability = one' indicates that an event is bound to occur.

Probability density: the scale of measurement on the *y*-axis used for all theoretical frequency distribution curves.

Quartiles: the values which occur in an ordered data set at the points which divide the whole range into four equal portions.

Random: occurring by chance.

Random number: a number selected by chance so that its value could not be predicted and there is no discernable pattern in any sequence of such numbers.

Random sampling: a sampling method that takes place without bias where each item in the sampling frame has an equal and independent chance of being selected as part of the sample.

Range: this is a measure of dispersion; it is the difference between the lowest and highest values in a set of data. Alternatively it is the 'whole set' of values, viewed as an ordered set.

Ratio measure: this is the highest and most precise level of measurement. The values of a variable can be differentiated, meaningfully ordered, the differences between them are assumed to be quantitatively equal, and the 'zero measure' is fixed – with an intrinsic meaning with respect to that variable.

Receiver operating characteristic: a combined measure of sensitivity and specificity which is used to examine the 'trade off' between sensitivity and specificity, for example in the value of a clinical test.

Regression: a procedure for working out the precise relationship between variables which can be used to predict the value of a dependent variable from that of an independent variable.

Relative frequency: the frequency of a particular value of a variable divided by the total frequency of all the values.

Relative risk: the ratio of the probabilities of an event occurring in two groups which each receive different treatments.

Sample: a set of individuals, units or items drawn from a population.

Sampling distribution: a theoretical distribution of statistics, such as sample means, from all possible samples of a given size taken from a population.

Sampling frame: a list of all the individuals, units or items in the population, from which a sample can be drawn.

Sampling procedure: a method used to obtain a sample from a population.

Sampling unit: an individual item of a population to be sampled.

Scatter diagram: a graph where each point plotted has its pair of coordinates being a pair of values of (possibly connected) variables.

Scatter plot: see Scatter diagram.

Sector: a portion of a circle bounded by two radii and an arc – a 'slice' of a circle.

Sensitivity: this measures the ability of a test to give a positive result in the presence of the condition in question. For example, in a sample of people who *in fact are* suffering from a particular disease, it is calculated as the ratio of the number who 'test positive' to the whole sample size.

Sign test: this is a non-parametric test which can be used instead of the paired t-test. It involves taking paired items of data and noting down the sign (+ or −) of the difference in each case. A binomial test is applied to the resulting numbers of '+s' and '−s'.

Significance level: this gives the probability that a valid null hypothesis would be rejected.

Significance test: a test to establish whether a null hypothesis should be accepted or rejected.

Skew: the extent to which an asymmetric frequency distribution has one of its 'tails' stretching out further than the other.

Spearman's correlation coefficient ('ρ', 'rho'): this is a non-parametric measure of correlation.

Specificity: this measures the ability of a test to give a negative result in the absence of the condition in question. For example, in a sample of people who *in fact are not* suffering from a particular disease, it is calculated as the ratio of the number who 'test negative' to the whole sample size.

Standard deviation: this is a very common measure of dispersion. The standard deviation of a sample is denoted by 's' and it is based on the average of the squares of the differences between the values of the variable and the sample mean. The standard deviation of a population is denoted by 'σ'.

Standard error of the mean: this is the standard deviation of the frequency distribution of sample means.

Standard error: a shortened form of 'Standard error of the mean'

Standard normal curve: the curve of the standard normal distribution.

Standard normal distribution: the normal distribution which has a mean of zero and a standard deviation of one.

Standard score: see z-score.

Standardise: to transform a value from any normal distribution (using a z-score) so that it belongs to the standard normal distribution.

Statistic: a quantity such as mean ($\bar{x}$), variance (s^2) or standard deviation (s) which characterises a sample.

Statistics: the whole subject involved with collecting and analysing real-life data, to summarise it and to display it, also to draw inferences from it to assist decision making.

Statistical significance: when a finding is significant at the 5% level, then it is 95% probable that the finding is not just a 'by chance'.

Stratified sampling: a sampling method which takes a random sample from each of the identified subsets (known as strata) of the population. Each stratum is sampled in proportion to its size.

Summary statistics: this is the term used for the individual numbers (such as mean and standard deviation) which summarise a data set.

Systematic sampling: a sampling method which selects units for the sample when they are 'equally spaced' in the sample frame, for example taking every 5th or 10th person from a list.

Tally chart: a simple chart on which a tick or stroke represents each occurrence of the value of a variable.

t-score: a transformed value from a distribution which may be normal but there is insufficient data to be sure of calculating a z-score.

t-test: a hypothesis test depending on the use of a t-score. There are three versions of the t-test, known as independent, paired and one sample t-tests.

Tukey's honestly significant difference test: a *post hoc* test used in analysis of variance to isolate differences between the groups but avoiding type I errors associated with multiple testing.

Two-tailed test: this is applied in the situation of a hypothesis test where the expectation is even handed – either the null hypothesis is valid or it is not valid.

Type I error: rejecting a null hypothesis even when it is valid and should be accepted.

Type II error: accepting a null hypothesis when it is not valid and should be rejected.

Uncertainty: the extent to which something cannot be known definitely.

Uni-dimensional scale: a rating scale (like a visual analogue scale) which measures only one dimension of a particular phenomenon, for example, intensity of pain.

Unimodal: a frequency distribution where there is a single value which uniquely has the maximum frequency.

Upper class boundary: the upper boundary of a class (or set) of grouped values of a variable. Any value greater than this must be in the next class.

Variable: any quality of interest that is likely to vary in different circumstances and different cases, for example weight, nationality.

Variance: this is a measure of dispersion; it is the square of the standard deviation.

Visual analogue scale: an interval scale on which a phenomenon, for example the intensity of pain, can be subjectively scored.

Wilcoxon signed-rank test: this is a non-parametric test which gives results similar to those of the Mann-Whitney U test.

Yate's correction (or Yate's continuity correction): this is a mathematical correction used to improve the accuracy of a chi-squared test when it is based on a '2 × 2' contingency table. It is advisable to apply this correction especially when the 'expected values' are small, that is, less than five.

z-score: a value from a normal distribution transformed by subtracting the population mean and dividing by the population standard deviation. The result is a value from the standard normal distribution.

Appendix 4

The ANOVA Estimates for Variance

(a) The within-sample estimate for σ^2 (see Section 10.3)

For sample A, we combine the expressions for s_A^2 and σ^2:

$$\sigma 2 = \frac{n}{n-1} \times \frac{\Sigma(x - \overline{x_A})^2}{n} \times \frac{\Sigma(x - \overline{x_A})^2}{n-1}$$

which can be written as $\Sigma(x - \overline{x_A})^2 = (n-1)\,\sigma^2$

Similarly for sample B and sample C we can write:

$$\Sigma(x - \overline{x_B})^2 = (n-1)\,\sigma^2 \quad \text{and} \quad \Sigma(x - \overline{x_C})^2 = (n-1)\,\sigma^2$$

Adding these together gives

$$\Sigma(x - \overline{x_A})^2 + \Sigma(x - \overline{x_B})^2 + \Sigma(x - \overline{x_C})^2 = (n-1)\,\sigma^2 + (n-1)\,\sigma^2 + (n-1)\,\sigma^2$$
$$= 3(n-1)\,\sigma^2$$

from which we get the overall within-sample estimate for σ^2

(b) The between-sample estimate for σ^2 (see Section 10.3)

An estimate for the variance of sample means is $\dfrac{\sigma^2}{n}$

We also have the variance of sample means $= \dfrac{\Sigma(\bar{x} - \bar{X})^2}{3 - 1}$

where $\bar{x}$ takes each of the values $\overline{x_A}$, $\overline{x_B}$, and $\overline{x_C}$ in turn.
   (We use '3 – 1' instead of '3' because we are estimating for a 'population of samples' from a (small) 'sample of samples'.).

We combine these expressions for variance to give: $\dfrac{\sigma^2}{n} = \dfrac{\Sigma(\bar{x} - \bar{X})^2}{3 - 1}$

from which we get the between-sample estimate for σ^2.

Appendix 5

Statistical Tables

(a) Random numbers (see Section 3.3)

233	630	406	791	916	656	461	771	607
653	576	710	887	871	103	937	705	938
274	017	381	454	446	567	278	436	545
935	535	338	970	706	601	352	120	178
490	028	884	846	460	056	635	406	267
838	158	240	292	921	106	257	966	306
529	452	847	979	794	480	268	092	743
852	395	466	917	176	761	287	101	761
899	067	406	539	395	588	037	338	678
908	260	615	644	440	109	435	531	295
388	510	316	956	560	033	799	643	257
564	816	628	670	703	374	741	649	842
869	048	288	886	867	772	255	576	078
212	229	680	048	481	142	578	506	258
331	286	405	112	128	829	312	236	987
535	140	770	350	503	387	947	625	545
557	723	595	359	595	501	652	643	812
895	648	319	840	408	786	640	343	021
694	388	392	747	479	945	227	974	795
961	175	057	183	831	167	921	401	963
578	819	634	940	403	305	565	207	958
942	767	739	891	918	962	704	497	216
317	052	862	110	102	278	332	948	867
982	532	882	416	163	396	749	653	822
720	700	737	095	952	261	994	619	084
809	957	593	608	080	023	108	809	207
687	383	702	056	569	916	961	816	289
886	655	854	360	601	114	514	497	190
824	509	758	066	662	281	231	828	361
969	137	348	870	706	631	194	352	897
953	821	282	997	974	464	924	556	825
442	404	880	897	967	735	675	794	649
515	572	118	891	915	531	038	990	421
012	138	196	020	204	423	903	076	454
612	934	881	850	504	419	749	283	866
897	423	638	566	664	437	713	086	068
742	728	166	372	723	342	342	338	752
067	877	924	343	435	469	236	218	807
905	794	305	564	642	231	976	504	719
664	580	551	075	750	057	829	884	483
515	068	814	433	332	225	575	858	569
376	602	257	650	509	897	327	262	220
804	290	904	220	205	506	316	156	644
209	734	805	702	028	827	096	770	050
980	450	545	940	406	605	640	391	121
422	065	998	130	310	079	190	125	157
599	735	913	616	168	809	921	475	261

Generated using Microsoft Office Excel 2003

(b) The standard normal distribution (see Section 6.4)

This table shows *right-hand tails* for the normal distribution N(0,1). Each z-score is used correct to two decimal places: the first place is read *down* the left column, the second is read *across* that row. The number from the table gives the proportion of the whole area beneath the curve which lies *to the right* of a vertical line through the z-score, that is, the probability of a score *greater than* that given. (NB. For a *negative* z, the number gives the *left-hand* tail.)

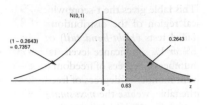

z	0	1	2	3	4	5	6	7	8	9
0.0	0.5000	0.4960	0.4920	0.4880	0.4840	0.4801	0.4761	0.4721	0.4681	0.4641
0.1	0.4602	0.4562	0.4522	0.4483	0.4443	0.4404	0.4364	0.4325	0.4286	0.4247
0.2	0.4207	0.4168	0.4129	0.4090	0.4052	0.4013	0.3974	0.3936	0.3897	0.3859
0.3	0.3821	0.3783	0.3745	0.3707	0.3669	0.3632	0.3594	0.3557	0.3520	0.3483
0.4	0.3446	0.3409	0.3372	0.3336	0.3300	0.3264	0.3228	0.3192	0.3156	0.3121
0.5	0.3085	0.3050	0.3015	0.2981	0.2946	0.2912	0.2877	0.2843	0.2810	0.2776
0.6	0.2743	0.2709	0.2676	0.2643	0.2611	0.2578	0.2546	0.2514	0.2483	0.2451
0.7	0.2420	0.2389	0.2358	0.2327	0.2296	0.2266	0.2236	0.2206	0.2177	0.2148
0.8	0.2119	0.2090	0.2061	0.2033	0.2005	0.1977	0.1949	0.1922	0.1894	0.1867
0.9	0.1841	0.1814	0.1788	0.1762	0.1736	0.1711	0.1685	0.1660	0.1635	0.1611
1.0	0.1587	0.1562	0.1539	0.1515	0.1492	0.1469	0.1446	0.1423	0.1401	0.1379
1.1	0.1357	0.1335	0.1314	0.1292	0.1271	0.1251	0.1230	0.1210	0.1190	0.1170
1.2	0.1151	0.1131	0.1112	0.1093	0.1075	0.1056	0.1038	0.1020	0.1003	0.0985
1.3	0.0968	0.0951	0.0934	0.0918	0.0901	0.0885	0.0869	0.0853	0.0838	0.0823
1.4	0.0808	0.0793	0.0778	0.0764	0.0749	0.0735	0.0721	0.0708	0.0694	0.0681
1.5	0.0668	0.0655	0.0643	0.0630	0.0618	0.0606	0.0594	0.0582	0.0571	0.0559
1.6	0.0548	0.0537	0.0526	0.0516	0.0505	0.0495	0.0485	0.0475	0.0465	0.0455
1.7	0.0446	0.0436	0.0427	0.0418	0.0409	0.0401	0.0392	0.0384	0.0375	0.0367
1.8	0.0359	0.0351	0.0344	0.0336	0.0329	0.0322	0.0314	0.0307	0.0301	0.0294
1.9	0.0287	0.0281	0.0274	0.0268	0.0262	0.0256	0.0250	0.0244	0.0239	0.0233
2.0	0.0228	0.0222	0.0217	0.0212	0.0207	0.0202	0.0197	0.0192	0.0188	0.0183
2.1	0.0179	0.0174	0.0174	0.0166	0.0162	0.0158	0.0154	0.0150	0.0146	0.0143
2.2	0.0139	0.0136	0.0132	0.0129	0.0125	0.0122	0.0119	0.0116	0.0113	0.0110
2.3	0.0107	0.0104	0.0102	0.0099	0.0096	0.0094	0.0091	0.0089	0.0087	0.0084
2.4	0.0082	0.0080	0.0078	0.0075	0.0073	0.0071	0.0069	0.0068	0.0066	0.0064
2.5	0.0062	0.0060	0.0059	0.0057	0.0055	0.0054	0.0052	0.0051	0.0049	0.0048
2.6	0.0047	0.0045	0.0044	0.0043	0.0041	0.0040	0.0039	0.0038	0.0037	0.0036
2.7	0.0035	0.0034	0.0033	0.0032	0.0031	0.0030	0.0029	0.0028	0.0027	0.0026
2.8	0.0026	0.0025	0.0024	0.0023	0.0023	0.0022	0.0021	0.0021	0.0020	0.0019
2.9	0.0019	0.0018	0.0018	0.0017	0.0016	0.0016	0.0015	0.0015	0.0014	0.0014
3.0	0.0013	0.0013	0.0013	0.0012	0.0012	0.0011	0.0011	0.0011	0.0010	0.0010
3.1	0.0010	0.0009	0.0009	0.0009	0.0008	0.0008	0.0008	0.0008	0.0007	0.0007
3.2	0.0007	0.0007	0.0006	0.0006	0.0006	0.0006	0.0005	0.0005	0.0005	0.0005
3.3	0.0005	0.0005	0.0005	0.0004	0.0004	0.0004	0.0004	0.0004	0.0004	0.0003
3.4	0.0003	0.0003	0.0003	0.0003	0.0003	0.0003	0.0003	0.0003	0.0003	0.0002
3.5	0.0002	0.0002	0.0002	0.0002	0.0002	0.0002	0.0002	0.0002	0.0002	0.0002
3.6	0.0002	0.0002	0.0001	0.0001	0.0001	0.0001	0.0001	0.0001	0.0001	0.0001
3.7	0.0001	0.0001	0.0001	0.0001	0.0001	0.0001	0.0001	0.0001	0.0001	0.0001
3.8	0.0001	0.0001	0.0001	0.0001	0.0001	0.0001	0.0001	0.0001	0.0001	0.0001
3.9	0.0000	0.0000	0.0000	0.0000	0.0000	0.0000	0.0000	0.0000	0.0000	0.0000

Data from Perry R. Hinton: *Statistics Explained: A Guide for Social Science Students*, Routledge 1995, Figure A.1, p. 306.

(c) The t-distribution (see Section 9.4)

This table gives the t-score which bounds the critical region of the distribution. It is used for one tailed tests (*right-hand tail*) or two-tailed tests at 5% *or* 1% significance levels, taking account of the number of degrees of freedom (df). Where the relevant number of degrees of freedom is not shown in the table, we use the *next smallest* that does appear; so for df = 45, which is not shown, we use the value df = 40. When df is *very large* we use the ∞ (i.e. 'infinity') value, which gives figures equivalent to those given by the normal distribution.

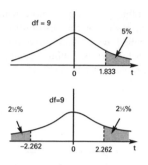

	0.05 Levels of significance		0.01 Level of significance	
df	One-tailed test	Two-tailed test	One-tailed test	Two-tailed test
1	6.314	12.706	31.821	63.657
2	2.920	4.303	6.965	9.925
3	2.353	3.182	4.541	5.841
4	2.132	2.776	3.747	4.604
5	2.015	2.571	3.365	4.032
6	1.943	2.447	3.143	3.707
7	1.895	2.365	2.998	3.499
8	1.860	2.306	2.896	3.355
9	1.833	2.262	2.821	3.250
10	1.812	2.228	2.764	3.169
11	1.796	2.201	2.718	3.106
12	1.782	2.179	2.681	3.055
13	1.771	2.160	2.650	3.012
14	1.761	2.145	2.624	2.977
15	1.753	2.131	2.602	2.947
16	1.746	2.120	2.583	2.921
17	1.740	2.110	2.567	2.898
18	1.734	2.101	2.552	2.878
19	1.729	2.093	2.539	2.861
20	1.725	2.086	2.528	2.845
21	1.721	2.080	2.518	2.831
22	1.717	2.074	2.508	2.819
23	1.714	2.069	2.500	2.807
24	1.711	2.064	2.492	2.797
25	1.708	2.060	2.485	2.787
26	1.706	2.056	2.479	2.779
27	1.703	2.052	2.473	2.771
28	1.701	2.048	2.467	2.763
29	1.699	2.045	2.462	2.756
30	1.697	2.042	2.457	2.750
40	1.684	2.021	2.423	2.704
60	1.671	2.000	2.390	2.660
120	1.658	1.980	2.358	2.617
∞	1.645	1.960	2.326	2.576

Data from Perry R. Hinton: *Statistics Explained: A Guide for Social Science Students*, Routledge, 1995; Figure A.2, p. 307.

(d) The chi-squared (χ^2) distribution (see Section 11.3)

This table gives the χ^2-score which bounds the critical region of the distribution. It is used for one tailed tests (*right-hand tail*) at 5% or 1% significance levels, taking account of the number of degrees of freedom (df).

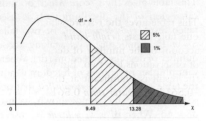

df	0.05 Level of significance	0.01 Level of significance
1	3.84	6.64
2	5.99	9.21
3	7.82	11.34
4	9.49	13.28
5	11.07	15.09
6	12.59	16.81
7	14.07	18.48
8	15.51	20.09
9	16.92	21.67
10	18.31	23.21
11	19.68	24.72
12	21.03	26.22
13	22.36	27.69
14	23.68	29.14
15	25.00	30.58
16	26.30	32.00
17	27.59	33.41
18	28.87	34.80
19	30.14	36.19
20	31.41	37.57
21	32.67	38.93
22	33.92	40.29
23	35.17	41.64
24	36.42	42.98
25	37.65	44.31
26	38.88	45.64
27	40.11	46.97
28	41.34	48.28
29	42.56	49.59
30	43.77	50.89

Data from Perry R. Hinton: *Statistics Explained: A Guide for Social Science Students*, Routledge, 1995; Figure A.7, p. 314.

(e) Pearson's correlation coefficient (r) (see Section 12.5)

This table gives the r-score which bounds the critical region of the distribution. It is used for one tailed tests (*right-hand tail*) or two-tailed tests at 5% or 1% significance levels, taking account of the number of degrees of freedom (df). df is always 'n – 2', the number of pairs of observations less two. Eg: with df = 6 in a one-tailed test, if r is greater than 0.6215 then the result is 'significant at the 5% level'; with df = 18 in a two-tailed test, if r is *less than* –0.5614 *or greater than* 0.5614 then the result is 'significant at the 1% level'.

df	0.05 Level of significance		0.01 Level of significance	
	One-tailed test (directional)	Two-tailed test (non-directional)	One-tailed test (directional)	Two-tailed test (non-directional)
1	0.9877	0.9969	0.9995	0.9999
2	0.9000	0.9500	0.9800	0.9900
3	0.8054	0.8783	0.9343	0.9587
4	0.7293	0.8114	0.8822	0.9172
5	0.6694	0.7545	0.8329	0.8745
6	0.6215	0.7067	0.7887	0.8343
7	0.5822	0.6664	0.7498	0.7977
8	0.5494	0.6319	0.7155	0.7646
9	0.5214	0.6021	0.6851	0.7348
10	0.4973	0.5760	0.6581	0.7079
11	0.4762	0.5529	0.6339	0.6835
12	0.4575	0.5324	0.6120	0.6614
13	0.4409	0.5139	0.5923	0.6411
14	0.4259	0.4973	0.5742	0.6226
15	0.4124	0.4821	0.5577	0.6055
16	0.4000	0.4683	0.5425	0.5897
17	0.3887	0.4555	0.5285	0.5751
18	0.3783	0.4438	0.5155	0.5614
19	0.3687	0.4329	0.5034	0.5487
20	0.3598	0.4227	0.4921	0.5368
25	0.3233	0.3809	0.4451	0.4869
30	0.2960	0.3494	0.4093	0.4487
35	0.2746	0.3246	0.3810	0.4182
40	0.2573	0.3044	0.3578	0.3932
45	0.2428	0.2875	0.3384	0.3721
50	0.2306	0.2732	0.3218	0.3541
60	0.2108	0.2500	0.2948	0.3248
70	0.1954	0.2319	0.2737	0.3017
80	0.1829	0.2172	0.2565	0.2830
90	0.1726	0.2050	0.2422	0.2673
100	0.1638	0.1946	0.2301	0.2540

Data from Perry R. Hinton: *Statistics Explained: A Guide for Social Science Students*, Routledge, 1995; Figure A.9, p. 316.

(f) Spearman's rank-correlation coefficient (ρ) (see Section 12.6)

This table gives the ρ-score which bounds the critical region of the distribution. It is used for one tailed tests (*right-hand tail*) or two-tailed tests at 5% or 1% significance levels, taking account of the number of categories, n i.e. the number of pairs of observations. Eg: with n = 7 in a one-tailed test, if ρ is greater than 0.714 then the result is 'significant at the 5% level'; with n = 12 in a two-tailed test, if ρ is *less than* –0.777 *or greater than* 0.777 then the result is 'significant at the 1% level'.

n	0.05 Level of significance		0.01 Level of significance	
	One-tailed test (directional)	Two-tailed test (non-directional)	One-tailed test (directional)	Two-tailed test (non-directional)
5	0.900	1.000	1.000	–
6	0.829	0.886	0.943	1.000
7	0.714	0.786	0.893	0.929
8	0.643	0.783	0.833	0.881
9	0.600	0.683	0.783	0.833
10	0.564	0.648	0.746	0.794
12	0.506	0.591	0.712	0.777
14	0.456	0.544	0.645	0.715
16	0.425	0.506	0.601	0.665
18	0.399	0.475	0.564	0.625
20	0.377	0.450	0.534	0.591
22	0.359	0.428	0.508	0.562
24	0.343	0.409	0.485	0.537
26	0.329	0.392	0.465	0.515
28	0.317	0.377	0.448	0.496
30	0.306	0.364	0.432	0.478

Data from Perry R. Hinton: *Statistics Explained: A Guide for Social Science Students*, Routledge, 1995; Figure A.10, p. 317.

(g) The F-distribution (see Section 10.3)

These two tables give the F-score which bounds the critical region of the distribution, at different levels of significance. They are used for one-tailed tests (*right hand tail*) only. The F-score is calculated as a fraction, and the values in the tables depend both on df1 (the number of degrees of freedom for the numerator, the top of the fraction) and on df2 (the number of degrees of freedom for the denominator, the bottom of the fraction). When the calculated F-score is *greater than* the value from the table, then the result is significant (at that % level).

0.05 Level of significance

df2	1	2	3	4	5	6	7	8	9	10	20	∞
1	161.45	199.50	215.71	224.58	230.16	233.99	236.77	238.88	240.54	241.88	248.01	254.32
2	18.51	19.00	19.16	19.25	19.30	19.35	19.33	19.37	19.38	19.40	19.45	19.50
3	10.13	9.55	9.28	9.12	9.01	8.94	8.89	8.85	8.81	8.79	8.66	8.53
4	7.71	6.94	6.59	6.39	6.26	6.16	6.09	6.04	6.00	5.96	5.80	5.63
5	6.61	5.79	5.41	5.19	5.05	4.95	4.88	4.82	4.77	4.74	4.56	4.36
6	5.99	5.14	4.76	4.53	4.39	4.28	4.21	4.15	4.10	4.06	3.87	3.67
7	5.59	4.74	4.35	4.12	3.97	3.87	3.79	3.73	3.68	3.64	3.44	3.23
8	5.32	4.46	4.07	3.84	3.69	3.58	3.50	3.44	3.39	3.35	3.15	2.93
9	5.12	4.26	3.86	3.63	3.48	3.37	3.29	3.23	3.18	3.14	2.94	2.71
10	4.96	4.10	3.71	3.48	3.33	3.22	3.14	3.07	3.02	2.98	2.77	2.54
11	4.84	3.98	3.59	3.36	3.20	3.09	3.01	2.95	2.90	2.85	2.65	2.40
12	4.75	3.89	3.49	3.26	3.11	3.00	2.91	2.85	2.80	2.75	2.54	2.30
13	4.67	3.81	3.41	3.18	3.03	2.92	2.83	2.77	2.71	2.67	2.46	2.21
14	4.60	3.74	3.34	3.11	2.96	2.85	2.76	2.70	2.65	2.60	2.39	2.13
15	4.54	3.68	3.29	3.06	2.90	2.79	2.71	2.64	2.59	2.54	2.33	2.07
16	4.49	3.63	3.24	3.01	2.85	2.74	2.66	2.59	2.54	2.49	2.28	2.01
17	4.45	3.59	3.20	2.96	2.81	2.70	2.61	2.55	2.49	2.45	2.23	1.96
18	4.41	3.55	3.16	2.93	2.77	2.66	2.58	2.51	2.46	2.41	2.19	1.92
19	4.38	3.52	3.13	2.90	2.74	2.63	2.54	2.48	2.42	2.38	2.16	1.88
20	4.35	3.49	3.10	2.87	2.71	2.60	2.51	2.45	2.39	2.35	2.12	1.84
21	4.32	3.47	3.07	2.84	2.68	2.57	2.49	2.42	2.37	2.32	2.10	1.81
22	4.30	3.44	3.05	2.82	2.66	2.55	2.46	2.40	2.34	2.30	2.07	1.78
23	4.28	3.42	3.03	2.80	2.64	2.53	2.44	2.37	2.32	2.27	2.05	1.76
24	4.26	3.40	3.01	2.78	2.62	2.51	2.42	2.36	2.30	2.25	2.03	1.73
25	4.24	3.39	2.99	2.76	2.60	2.49	2.40	2.34	2.28	2.24	2.01	1.71
26	4.23	3.37	2.98	2.74	2.59	2.47	2.39	2.32	2.27	2.22	1.99	1.69
27	4.21	3.35	2.96	2.73	2.57	2.46	2.37	2.31	2.25	2.20	1.97	1.67
28	4.20	3.34	2.95	2.71	2.56	2.45	2.36	2.29	2.24	2.19	1.96	1.65
29	4.18	3.33	2.93	2.70	2.55	2.43	2.35	2.28	2.22	2.18	1.94	1.64
30	4.17	3.32	2.92	2.69	2.53	2.42	2.33	2.27	2.21	2.16	1.93	1.62
40	4.08	3.23	2.84	2.61	2.45	2.34	2.25	2.18	2.12	2.08	1.84	1.51
60	4.00	3.15	2.76	2.53	2.37	2.25	2.17	2.10	2.04	1.99	1.75	1.39
120	3.92	3.07	2.68	2.45	2.29	2.18	2.09	2.02	1.96	1.91	1.66	1.25
∞	3.84	3.00	2.60	2.37	2.21	2.10	2.01	1.94	1.88	1.83	1.57	1.00

0.01 Level of significance

df2	*df1* 1	2	3	4	5	6	7	8	9	10	20	∞
1	4052.2	4999.5	5403.3	5624.6	5763.7	5859.0	5928.3	5981.6	6022.5	6055.8	6208.7	6366.0
2	98.50	99.00	99.17	99.25	99.30	99.33	99.36	99.37	99.39	99.40	99.45	99.50
3	34.12	30.82	29.46	28.71	28.24	27.91	27.67	27.49	27.34	27.23	26.69	26.12
4	21.20	18.00	16.69	15.98	15.52	15.21	14.98	14.80	14.66	14.55	14.02	13.46
5	16.26	13.27	12.06	11.39	10.97	10.67	10.46	10.29	10.16	10.05	9.55	9.02
6	13.74	10.92	9.78	9.15	8.75	8.47	8.26	8.10	7.98	7.87	7.40	6.88
7	12.25	9.55	8.45	7.85	7.46	7.19	6.99	6.84	6.72	6.62	6.16	5.65
8	11.26	8.65	7.59	7.01	6.63	6.37	6.18	6.03	5.91	5.81	5.36	4.86
9	10.56	8.02	6.99	6.42	6.06	5.80	5.61	5.47	5.35	5.26	4.81	4.31
10	10.04	7.56	6.55	5.99	5.64	5.39	5.20	5.06	4.94	4.85	4.41	3.91
11	9.65	7.21	6.22	5.67	5.32	5.07	4.89	4.74	4.63	4.54	4.10	3.60
12	9.33	6.93	5.95	5.41	5.06	4.82	4.64	4.50	4.39	4.30	3.86	3.36
13	9.07	6.70	5.74	5.21	4.86	4.62	4.44	4.30	4.19	4.10	3.66	3.17
14	8.86	6.51	5.56	5.04	4.70	4.46	4.28	4.14	4.03	3.94	3.51	3.00
15	8.68	6.36	5.42	4.89	4.56	4.32	4.14	4.00	3.89	3.80	3.37	2.87
16	8.53	6.23	5.29	4.77	4.44	4.20	4.03	3.89	3.78	3.69	3.26	2.75
17	8.40	6.11	5.18	4.67	4.34	4.10	3.93	3.79	3.68	3.59	3.16	2.65
18	8.29	6.01	5.09	4.58	4.25	4.01	3.84	3.71	3.60	3.51	3.08	2.57
19	8.18	5.93	5.01	4.50	4.17	3.94	3.77	3.63	3.52	3.43	3.00	2.49
20	8.10	5.85	4.94	4.43	4.10	3.87	3.70	3.56	3.46	3.37	2.94	2.42
21	8.02	5.78	4.87	4.37	4.04	3.81	3.64	3.51	3.40	3.31	2.88	2.36
22	7.95	5.72	4.82	4.31	3.99	3.76	3.59	3.45	3.35	3.26	2.83	2.31
23	7.88	5.66	4.76	4.26	3.94	3.71	3.54	3.41	3.30	3.21	2.78	2.26
24	7.82	5.61	4.72	4.22	3.90	3.67	3.50	3.36	3.26	3.17	2.74	2.21
25	7.77	5.57	4.68	4.18	2.86	3.86	3.63	3.46	3.32	3.22	2.70	2.17
26	7.72	5.53	4.64	4.14	3.82	3.59	3.42	3.29	3.18	3.09	2.66	2.13
27	7.68	5.49	4.60	4.11	3.78	3.56	3.39	3.26	3.15	3.06	2.63	2.10
28	7.64	5.45	4.57	4.07	3.75	3.53	3.36	3.23	3.12	3.03	2.60	2.06
29	7.60	5.42	4.54	4.04	3.73	3.50	3.33	3.20	3.09	3.00	2.57	2.03
30	7.56	5.39	4.51	4.02	3.70	3.47	3.30	3.17	3.07	2.98	2.55	2.01
40	7.31	5.18	4.31	3.83	3.51	3.29	3.12	2.99	2.89	2.80	2.37	1.80
60	7.08	4.98	4.13	3.65	3.34	3.12	2.95	2.82	2.72	2.63	2.20	1.60
120	6.85	4.79	3.95	3.48	3.17	2.96	2.79	2.66	2.56	2.47	2.03	1.38
∞	6.63	4.61	3.78	3.32	3.02	2.80	2.64	2.51	2.41	2.32	1.88	1.00

Data from Perry R. Hinton: *Statistics Explained: A Guide for Social Science Students*, Routledge, 1995; Figure A.3 pp. 308–9.

Index

Note: Page numbers in **bold** refer to entries in the Glossary.